# Praise for

# ***"The Journey to Black Belt"***

Kevin Brett's book is the perfect book for anyone who is interested in getting into the martial arts or getting their children started in the martial arts. *The Journey to Black Belt* covers everything that a potential student needs to know in order to make an informed decision when it comes to selecting the right martial arts style, school, and instructor. He explains the difference in the individual martial arts, as well as guides the reader concerning what he or she should look for when trying to decide on the right instructor. Mr. Brett even covers things such as discovering your true goals and how to achieve your goals.

The book is organized much like an outline with short topic sections throughout. I personally find books which are formatted in this style, especially guide books or resource books, much easier to read and follow. The format and style of this book is perfect. This is, without a doubt, the most complete book of its kind on the market. I really can't think of anything that a potential martial arts student would need to know that *The Journey to Black Belt* leaves out. It is simply that complete!

Bohdi Sanders, Ph.D.
Author:
***Wisdom of the Elders,***
***Wicked Wisdom: Explorations into the Dark Side,***
***Life Lessons: Politically Incorrect Wisdom,***
***Fireside Meditations***
*www.TheWisdomWarrior.com*

*The Journey to Black Belt*

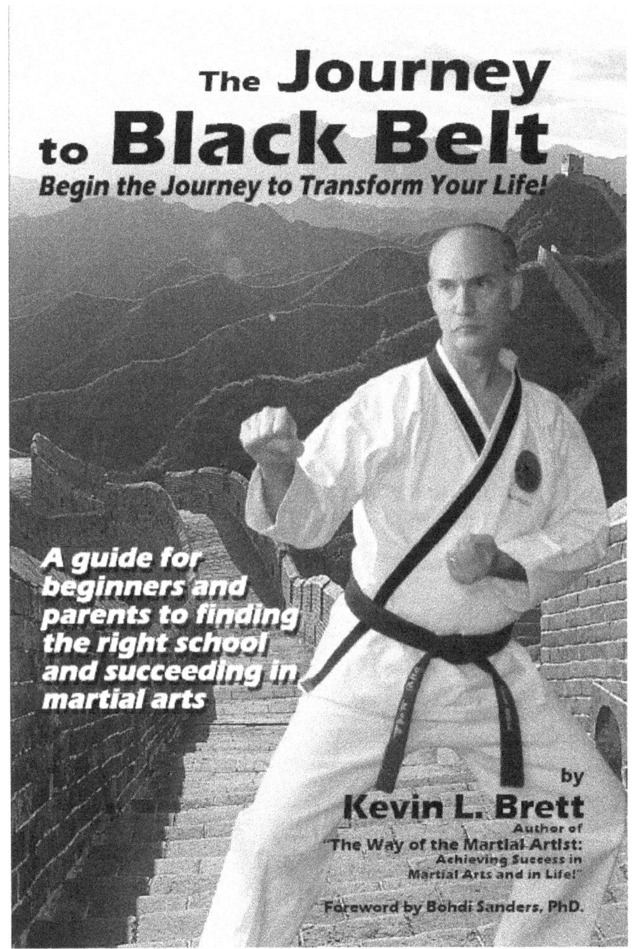


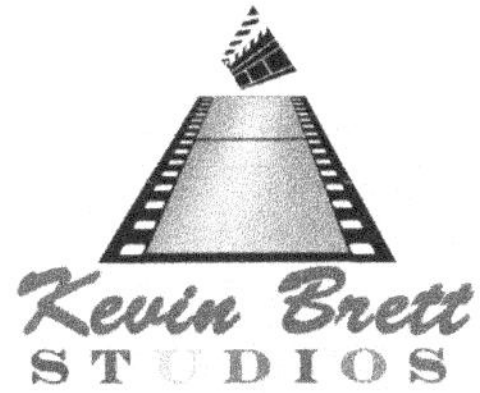


**Entertainment | Education | Family**

**www.KevinBrettStudios.com**

This book includes information from many sources and gathered from many personal experiences. It is published for general reference and is not intended to be a substitute for qualified martial arts instruction or expert instruction and advice, or medical advice. This book is sold with the understanding that neither the author nor the publisher is engaged in rendering legal, psychological, medical or other advice related to the topics referenced in this book. The publisher and author disclaim any personal liability, directly or indirectly, for advice or information presented within. Although the author and publisher have prepared this manuscript with utmost care and diligence and have made every effort to ensure the accuracy and completeness of the information contained within, we assume no responsibility for errors, inaccuracies omissions or inconsistencies.

**Publisher's Cataloging-In-Publication Data**
(Prepared by The Donohue Group, Inc.)

Brett, Kevin L.
The Journey to Black Belt: Begin the Journey to Transform Your Life! / Kevin L. Brett.

p. : ill. ; cm.

Includes index.
ISBN-13: 978-0981935041
ISBN-10: 0981935044

1. Martial arts--Psychological aspects. 2. Martial arts. 3. Self-realization. 4. Mind and body. I. Title.

GV1102.7.P75 B74 2011
796.8 2011911902

**ATTN: Quantity discounts are available to your company educational institution, government agency or martial arts organization.**

For more information, please contact the author at Kevin Brett Studios, Inc.
19 Live Oak Lane, Stafford, Virginia 22554 540-845-4755
sales@KevinBrettStudios.com

# Dedication

I dedicate this book to the spirit of those of you who want to transform your lives through your martial arts experience. Through hard work, sweat and a burning desire to excel in everything you do, you will gain confidence and daring on your Journey to Black Belt ... and beyond. May you embody the spirit of the servant warrior and give back to others some part of what you have been blessed with on your journey.

## A Warrior's Creed

*The journey of the warrior, for those sincere, is one*
*with many destinations; but mind,*
*body and spirit must be one.*
*It is in the fires of our will that we forge our*
*bodies and spirit to defend ourselves and protect others.*
*The warrior must always seek enlightenment and*
*live with honor and in service to others.*

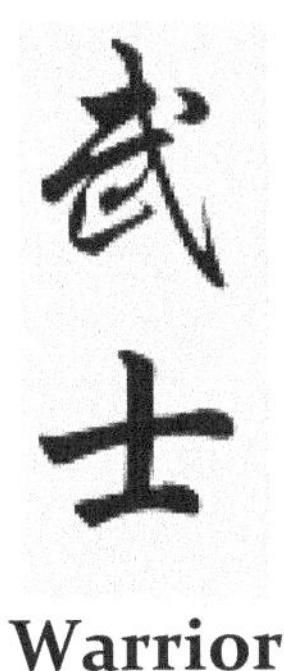


**Warrior**

# WARNING & DISCLAIMER

Marital arts can be lethal and the practice of martial arts or application of various martial arts techniques, training drills and exercises can cause serious injury or death. This book is intended for informational and entertainment purposes. It is not intended as a substitute for a specific martial arts training program by a qualified martial arts school or instructor. You should consult a qualified physician before engaging in any exercise program or physical activities to ascertain whether you or the other participants are mentally and physically healthy enough to engage in such activities.

Martial arts are for defensive purposes only and should be used only as a last resort and only with the least amount of force or technique necessary to reduce the immediate threat or risk in a self-defense situation. Anyone applying fighting or martial arts techniques or methods could be liable in civil or criminal court. You must control your actions and remain within the boundaries of the laws of the jurisdiction in which any defensive techniques may be employed.

The author, publisher and sellers of this book assume no liability for personal injury or damage to property as a result of practicing any concepts or content represented or implied within this book. All individuals are responsible for their own actions. The author, publisher and sellers of this book also provide no warranty or guarantee, expressed or implied that the techniques, concepts or content presented in this book will be effective in any or all self-defense situations.

## *Do You Have Everything You Need to Succeed in the Martial Arts and in Life?*

Kevin Brett Studios is the author of, the book, ***"The Way of the Martial Artist: Achieving Success in Martial Arts and in Life!"***

(240 pp., $11.95, ISBN-13: 978-0981935003), available from Amazon.com, Books.Google.com, BarnesandNobel.com in print or for Kindle or from the author's website www.KevinBrettStudios.com This book helps readers what is likely lacking in their training, and what it means to have a well-rounded martial arts education. Certified Martial Arts Instructor Kevin Brett provides insights into the origins, skills, training methods, strategies, tactics and character and spirit of the martial artist. This book is jammed with motivation, inspiration and education for martial artists from beginners to master-level and it culminates with the chapter: Success for Life which provides readers with seventeen techniques to incorporate in your training and your every day life to achieve your most important goals. It also covers the five elements of success and teaches you how to develop your own personal blueprint for translating the achievements, discipline and success factors you achieve in martial arts into every other aspect of your life!

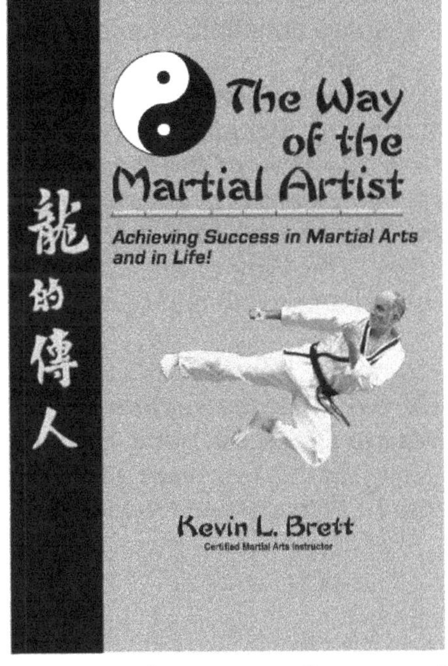


Martial arts are about survival and this book teaches readers how to develop the skill, strategy and character of a true martial artist to supplement their dojo training. It also provides in-depth insight into just what students and parents want from martial arts: discipline, commitment, honor, respect, perseverance and ultimately – success in any life-undertaking. Kevin Brett provides answers and insights to questions that all martial artists ask during their quest for excellence, purpose and enlightenment.

***The Way of the Martial Artist: Achieving Success in Martial Arts and in Life!*** uses the principles of martial arts to show readers how any worthwhile goal or life challenge can be approached and achieved with black belt determination. The servant-warrior is an ancient concept that the author re-introduces to help modern readers understand how any success should be a service or benefit to others.

Shawn Kovacich, author of the highly acclaimed book series ***Achieving Kicking Excellence*** and high-ranking martial artist, calls ***The Way of the Martial Artist***, *"A comprehensive framework of the numerous principles and concepts you will need to become the best martial artist that you can be."* Black belt Richard Hefner says, *"The Way of the Martial Artist is part success manual, part martial arts guide and part survival guide, and all essential!"*

Lawrence Kane, author of ***Surviving Armed Assaults*** and ***Martial Arts Instruction***; co-author of ***The Way of Kata***, ***The Way to Black Belt***, and The ***Little Black Book of Violence*** says, *"Kevin Brett has written an informative, interesting and useful book that I wholeheartedly recommend."*

# Contents

# *The Journey to Black Belt*

# Foreword

People become interested in martial arts for a variety of reasons. Some people find the traditions and mysteries of the martial arts intriguing and are interested in the martial arts strictly as an art form. Other people are interested in the sports aspect of the martial arts - competition in tournament sparring, forms or breaking. Many are looking for a way to instill positive character traits and self-esteem in their children. Others are only interested in pure self-defense and are not concerned with the art form, history, traditions, or competitions.

All of these are valid reasons to explore the world of martial arts, but becoming interested in the martial arts is only the first step. Deciding that you want to pursue your goals through the study of martial arts is the easy part; it is much harder to find the right dojo to train in and a qualified teacher. It is easy to be taken advantage of when you are entering into unfamiliar territory, especially if you have not taken the time to do your homework. This is where The Journey to Black Belt: A Beginner and Parent's Guide to Finding the Right School and Succeeding in Martial Arts comes into play.

Kevin Brett has put together a wonderful book that guides the novice through the sometimes confusing and foreign world of martial arts. The martial arts are no different than any other subject when it comes to doing your homework; you need to understand something about the subject before you jump in with both feet or, in the case of the martial arts, before you sign a contract.

Most people would not buy a new car without doing some research on the different types and models of cars that they are considering buying. They would compare prices, warranties, safety concerns, companies, etc. The same principle applies to finding the right martial arts dojo.

Today, more than ever before, the consumer has an enormous variety of choices when it comes to choosing a martial arts dojo or an instructor to guide them to the fulfillment of their goals in the martial arts. Furthermore, just as there are good restaurants and bad restaurants in every city and town across America, there are also good martial arts instructors and bad martial arts instructors. In addition, there is a wide variety of choices when it comes to different styles of martial arts, not to mention the different philosophies of the individual instructors.

To the novice, with no experience in the martial arts, the range of choices can be mind-boggling. The task of deciding on a martial arts school for the beginner, could be compared to someone walking into a gun shop to buy a gun with absolutely no experience or knowledge of firearms. Unless that person is very lucky, he is just asking to be taken advantage of by an unscrupulous owner. This is not wise.

Moreover, even for people who do take the time to research the martial arts, all of the bogus and conflicting information out there can make it a daunting task to filter through it all and decide which martial art is right for them. Even after deciding on a specific martial art that will help them with their personal goals, they still have the intimidating task of then finding a truly qualified instructor.

As you can see, there is much more involved in choosing the right dojo for your training than picking up the phone book and flipping through the yellow pages. But unfortunately, this is how the vast majority of people decide on martial arts school, and as a result, many people walk away from their experience in the martial arts disheartened and disappointed.

Although it is highly unlikely that you will find any martial arts school or instructor which is perfect in every way, there are some very important criteria that you should look for in choosing both the right school and the right instructor. By definition, the martial arts are about learning methods of self-defense. Learning to successfully defend yourself is at the core of what the martial arts are all about, although as I stated above, different people in today's society have different goals when it comes to the martial arts.

No matter what your own personal goals are where the martial arts are concerned, there are certain things that you should look for in making the various decisions concerning your training. Is the instructor truly experienced and qualified to help you meet your personal goals? Is the instructor's philosophy compatible with your own personal ethics? Is the instructor a man of honor and integrity or is he merely someone who knows how to fight? Is what the instructor teaches truly useful or is he simply teaching you rote punches and kicks which have no true value in the real world? These are just a sampling of the questions that you need to consider before you sign on that dotted line.

Your martial arts training should guide you on your journey to live the warrior lifestyle. This is what true martial arts are all about. Don't misunderstand me here. I'm not saying that the martial arts should lead you to a career in the military or in law enforcement. That is not what is meant by the warrior lifestyle.

The warrior lifestyle is a lifestyle of excellence, of character, of integrity, and of honor. The old martial arts masters knew this and considered this such an important consideration that they refused to instruct anyone whose character was suspect. The character of your instructor should be a primary focus when it comes to choosing the right martial arts dojo, especially if you are looking for a school for your children. Any martial arts school which neglects this part of a student's training is leaving out what should be one of your primary goals in studying the martial arts – the perfection of your character.

Gichin Funakoshi, the founder of Shotokan karate made this perfectly clear when he stated, "The ultimate aim of karate-do lies not in victory or defeat, but in the perfection of character of its participants." Ultimately, the perfection of one's character, and the ability to defend yourself and your loved ones, is what true martial arts and the warrior lifestyle is all about. The trick is to find the right instructor which understands this concept.

Kevin Brett has made the task of filtering through the perplexing amount of information available to the novice martial artist, much easier with this wonderfully complete book. The Journey to Black Belt: A Beginner and Parent's Guide to Finding the Right School and Succeeding in Martial Arts helps the reader decide what his or her ultimate goals are, which style of martial art is best for his or her goals, what to look for in a good school and a good instructor, and much more. This is the most complete book on the subject that I know of, and is sure to be a valuable resource for anyone who has the desire to start the rewarding journey to a black belt and beyond.

***Bohdi Sanders, Ph.D.***

*Bohdi Sanders is the author of the award winning Warrior Wisdom Series, the award winning* ***Wisdom of the Elders****,* ***Wicked Wisdom: Explorations into the Dark Side****,* ***Life Lessons: Politically Incorrect Wisdom****, and* ***Fireside Meditations****. He is also a member of the International Independent Martial Artist's Association Hall of Fame for his literary contributions to the martial arts with his Warrior Wisdom Series. His website, The Wisdom Warrior, can be found at: www.TheWisdomWarrior.com. Dr. Sanders may be reached by email at: WarriorWisdom@comcast.net*

# Introduction

*"Warriors are expected to be servants of society and people of virtue."*

My name is Kevin Brett. I am a certified Martial Arts Instructor with more than twenty years of training and teaching experience in the martial arts and the author of ***The Way of the Martial Artist: Achieving Success in Martial Arts and in Life!***

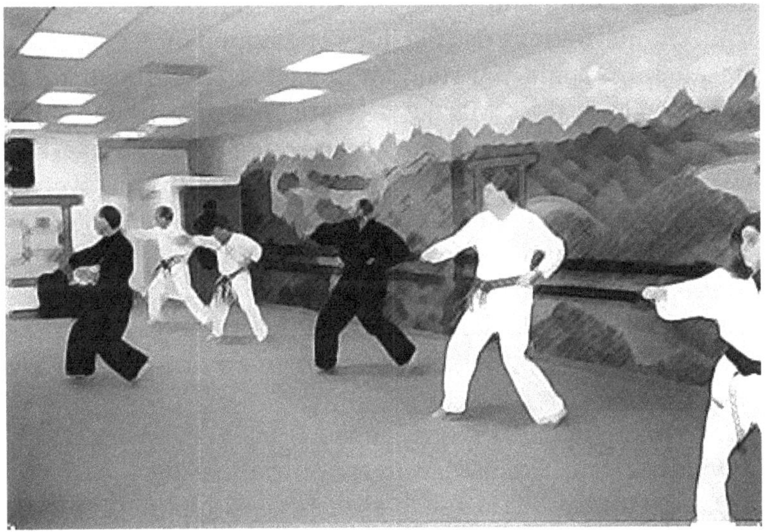

I have developed this new book *"**The Journey to Black Belt**"* to help beginning martial artists and you parents who are considering involving your children in the world of martial arts. My hope is that the ideas and information I share in these pages will help you to become more knowledgeable about martial arts, how to find a good school, understand what it takes to succeed in martial arts and in life and how martial arts study can change your life or your child's life for the better.

To the outsider, trying to understand and get started in martial arts can be confusing, mysterious and even frustrating. The information in this book will help you or your child get off to a great start in the exciting world of martial arts as you begin your journey to black belt. Shopping for a school involves understanding the benefits, how to know when you've found a good school and a style and how to sort your way through all the marketing and advertising hype. With the information in this book you can reap the rewards and enjoy martial arts to the fullest. I wish you much success!

Martial arts and the journey to black belt can be one of the most rewarding undertakings of your life. The confidence and character that result from achieving such an objective are difficult to match in any other endeavor. Martial arts are indeed a lifelong journey that can continue to provide endless rewards. Like life, martial arts present challenges and opportunities for growth. How we handle these challenges is key. If we handle them well, we will grow in character, stature and maturity and reach new levels of personal excellence. If we handle them poorly and do not learn the lessons that are there for us to experience, we risk stumbling down a path that can lead to frustration, disappointment and failure.

There are many benefits to be gained from martial arts study for both children and adults. Parents typically expect martial arts schools to instill key virtues such as respect, discipline, goal-setting, determination and of-course, self-defense and fitness. There are many styles of martial arts; many masters, many schools and many training methods from which to choose. There are also many different types of martial arts programs and memberships and payment plans. A little education in the whole matter will go a long way to helping you feel more confident in whatever decision you make.

I have designed this book to help the beginner understand four things:

- **Achieving Success in Martial Arts:** *What martial arts are all about and what it takes to be successful for children and adults*
- **Key Martial Arts Concepts:** *Training and defense concepts*
- **Martial Arts History and Styles:** *Evolution and the differences between the various styles*
- **Shopping for a School and Style of Martial Art:** *How to shop with confidence for a martial arts school and know what you're getting*

I have also built some useful appendices for your reference:

- Appendix A: Listing of major martial arts school directories on the internet
- Appendix B: Martial Arts Dictionary of common terms from various styles
- Appendix C: Goal Setting and Planning Worksheet

At the end of each chapter is a box titled "Resources". It contains excellent books on various aspects of martial arts. I highly recommend these books. I know many of the authors personally and they are among the most talented and knowledgeable martial artists in the dojo, on the street and in print! Check out their works and you will learn much.

I would also recommend you consider obtaining a copy of my book ***"The Way of the Martial Artist: Achieving Success in Martial Arts and in Life!"*** to accompany you as you begin your journey in the martial arts. Many notable martial artists have highly recommended it as an invaluable guide for martial artists at any experience level.

I hope the end result of reading this book is that you feel much more educated and confident about searching for a school. I hope the process of selecting a given style to study and the benefits you can expect from different training approaches becomes clearer and most importantly you understand how martial arts study, discipline and values can help enrich your life or your child's life so that you might transcend the martial arts experience and achieve success in every area of your life!

*Welcome to the martial arts.*
*Your journey to Black Belt and personal transformation begins now!*

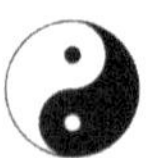

# Chapter 1

# *Succeeding in Martial Arts*

*"If you want to change your life, then you'll need to trade in your wishbone for a backbone and get started."*

**Dream | Commit | Achieve**

## *Purpose*

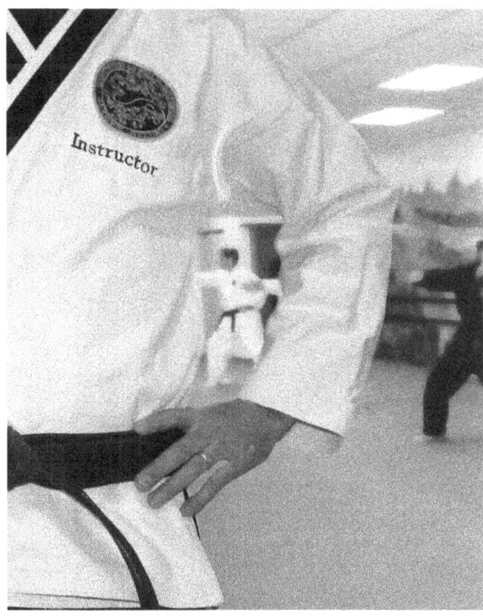


The original and continuing purpose of martial arts is to empower the individual. Martial arts are not intended only for the strong, but to strengthen the weak and provide them with alternatives to confront an aggressor. Your ultimate goal as a martial artist should be to pursue excellence in all life-endeavors and to serve as an example to others and use your new found skills, discipline and success secrets to find ways to give back to society.

I hope that through appreciation of the diversity of martial arts that students will learn to appreciate the diversity of peoples, cultures and society. Martial arts training can help strengthen tolerance, understanding and acceptance, the very qualities that are so important today and yet seem to be in such short supply.

To the novice or outsider, martial arts are just learning how to kick and punch. To a serious student or instructor it is much more. Martial arts is just that, an art; a means of expression. All martial arts are intended as a means of self-defense and are not intended for offensive purposes or antagonism. To violate this tenet is to violate the very essence of martial arts.

Serious martial artists should be concerned with history. Studying a series of moves or a set of forms serves little purpose if the student knows nothing of where the style derived, how the moves would realistically be applied or where the form originated and why.

Martial arts have a rich and fascinating history. There are hundreds of major styles of martial arts in existence today with Tae Kwon Do being the most widespread. Martial arts students should start by familiarizing themselves with the history and evolution of their own style. Eventually as a student climbs their way up the mountain to black belt level and beyond, they will, or should develop some familiarity with other styles and histories and differences between martial arts systems.

## *Tips for Parents*

Lot's of parents have found karate offers their children many benefits they cannot find in other athletic activities. In Chapter 2 ***Transforming Our Children's Character through Martial Arts***, I will give you a closer look at the character development and life-changing effects that can result from martial arts study. There are some other important insights parents need to ensure their children do well.

Martial arts do not happen overnight. Your child will not become a virtuoso pianist overnight, nor will they become a stellar black belt after a few weeks of lessons, but they will progress over time if they are committed. The first thing parents need to understand is that most people -- especially children -- are not able to train every day. Martial arts are like studying. The best results come from working at a steady pace -- not from cramming. Sports psychologists call this distributed practice versus massed practice. I call it common sense.

Most children will quickly tire of something if they do it every day. Martial arts are no exception. Parents help your children by fostering a training schedule that results in two or three lessons or classes every week. This kind of schedule prevents burnout. It gives the body a chance to rebuild properly. So, I encourage you to set a regular schedule that allows your child to progress steadily instead of cramming at the last minute. Hopefully this same concept will carry over into their school and studies as well. A good habit can be applied in multiple areas of life!

It's also important to get your child to class on time. This means wearing the uniform, or allowing a few extra minutes to change. Again, this will help them develop good habits of planning ahead and more effectively managing their time.

There are some other important tips that will help your child progress; one includes his or her uniform. Both the belt and the uniform deserve respect. In martial arts, the belt is a symbol of accomplishment, as well as rank. The uniform is a symbol of training and hard work. Children should not play in their uniforms and should treat their belt with respect. When they are in the Dojang, Dojo, or training hall, they must follow the rules of the school. This includes neat and clean dress.

Positive reinforcement is very important. When your child does something well, make a point of mentioning it. Always praise your child for his or her efforts. Praise encourages good performance and helps build the child's sense of self-esteem which is an essential ingredient to a happy and successful life.

Just as parent involvement is important in an academic setting, your interest and cooperation will speed your child's progress in martial arts. Again, it is important to remember that most things in life -- including martial arts -- require time and hard work to achieve mastery. There are no overnight wonders in the martial arts world.

Hard work, patience, praise, communication and cooperation will result in progress for your child. By helping our children reach their potential, we are improving the quality of life not just for them, but for everyone. Remember... they are the future!

## *Martial Arts Today*

Martial arts in the 21$^{st}$ century are concerned more with the practical application of techniques, sport and competition. However, martial arts study for adults and children has retained many of the core values of martial arts of old. The values associated with martial arts study are like the interwoven threads that hold society together. The values include respect, perseverance, self-discipline, self-respect, kindness, tolerance, honesty and loyalty.

Much of the deterioration, crime and moral decay in today's society can be directly linked to deterioration in core values. Where there is an absence of these values there are serious problems. Martial arts study and the pursuit of martial arts goals entails development and enhancement of these core values within the student. This system has been proven countless times to benefit children in their formative years and adults as well.

Martial arts students, whether child or adult, quickly learn the value of hard work, determination, honesty, and respect. They also learn many other qualities that are necessary for being happy with themselves and successful in their lives; that is a key theme in my book, ***"The Way of the Martial Artist: Achieving Success in Martial Arts and in Life!"*** In short, to study martial arts is to learn to be the master of oneself.

As a student, you will develop true self-confidence from accomplishing your goals in martial arts. You will learn the value of setting goals and maintaining consistent effort to accomplish them. That is a quality that will serve you or your child for a lifetime.

The confidence and character that many students develop is amazing and the transformation is for life. Often, they find that they are not easily tempted or influenced by peer pressure. Students learn to avoid rather than resort to violent solutions to problems and conflicts in their lives. With their newfound self-confidence many students are motivated to take on new challenges in their life. For some it may be beginning a new sport that they had never considered themselves able to handle. For others it may be taking on new challenges and roles of leadership and responsibility in their work, school or other career activities.

Martial arts is much more than simply kicking and punching; it is the development of the character and the improvement of self. Students improve their work or study habits and many students reach heights that they had never thought possible. Perseverance allows a student to continue to pass through levels of self-realization that would have never been possible otherwise. As I mentioned in ***"The Way of the Martial Artist"*** – *"To achieve your dreams, you must leave your comfort zone and never return."*

The lessons to be learned in martial arts continue to prove themselves to be just as important today as they were thousands of years ago. Through many centuries, martial arts have survived changes in government, culture and technology. They are as important today in the 21st century as they were long ago. Welcome to the martial arts. Train hard and enjoy!

## *Martial Arts Are About Survival*

Here's a shocker for you ... martial arts are about survival. Yep, that's right. The purpose of martial arts is to have the skill and knowledge to be able to do in the bad guy and still make it home in time to walk the dog. Martial arts are not some trendy type of workout designed to impress the ladies as you tell them about the tournaments or trophies you've won. While it certainly is an awesome total-body workout and a great way to get in shape, many students really give little thought to its ultimate purpose; survival.

Let's talk self-defense. I was one of the co-founders of the United Karate Institute of Self-Defense, Inc. in Alexandria, Virginia. Three other instructors, my wife (also a black belt) and I decided that we had met way too many highly ranked black belts who had earned numerous trophies in sport karate competition. They were champions and winners and knew all the tricks in the ring to score points and come home with the large gleaming plastic and marble trophies. Sounds great doesn't it. Except for one small problem, many of these black belt "champions" did not possess even the most basic skills or knowledge of how to defend themselves against even a single assailant, much less multiple assailants. What's up with that?

They're black belts. They should be able to leap over tall buildings, outrun bullets, stop a speeding train and run between the raindrops without getting wet! Right? No, but it certainly seems to the average person that a black belt must be nearly indestructible and probably possesses some almost mystical power and knowledge. Wrong again. If you are not trained properly with a real emphasis on effective, simple, proven self-defense and street application of martial arts techniques then you are merely mimicking movements from your instructor.

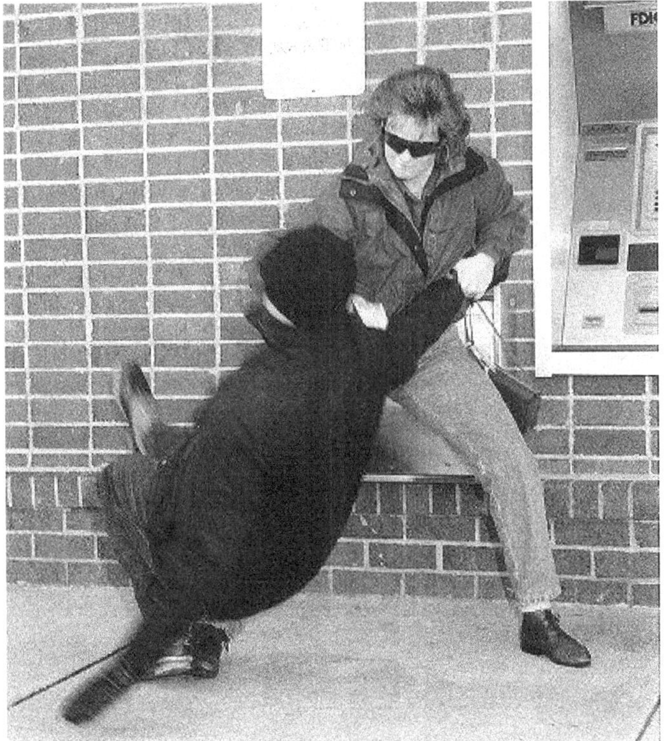


*If you can't defend yourself... nothing else matters!*

If you're a black belt and you can't even defend yourself on the street against common types of assaults then what have you spent all of those years doing? Let me say it again, ***martial arts are about survival.*** It's not about phony point-sparring competition where the only techniques you can use in the ring are things you would never dream of using on the street and where the most effective techniques from the street are not allowed in the ring. If your teenage daughter is taking martial arts, wouldn't you want her to really learn the effective close-quarters combatives that police and the military use to defend themselves and subdue attackers? It's all martial arts and effective techniques do not require one to be built like an NFL linebacker for them to work.

When you study martial arts it's not all just punching and kicking, you must learn about many qualities of humanity, both positive and negative because your brain is your ultimate survival tool. Among these qualities are determination, patience, balance, humility, respect, service, and even compassion. Ultimately, at its core, is the need to survive; be it on the streets of New York City, the jungles of Asia, the deserts of the Middle East or even a hostile work environment. To survive combat and harsh environments, you the martial artist must have many skills and have developed many physical and character qualities. However, remember the best warrior is not warlike, but is able to summon the warrior spirit within when it is required. It is a life-long journey.

## *A Mindset for Success*

There is more to martial arts and the pursuit of human excellence than simply working up a good sweat. We all wish to realize our potential in many endeavors in our life's journey. Through martial arts, your potential for human development is unlimited. Success is about constantly sculpting and shaping yourself until reality matches your dreams. What I am talking about when we discuss success is what you plan to make of the future. What will today hold? How will it bring you closer to your goals and what will you do to become excellent?

A martial art is a system of self-improvement on many levels, not merely a library of techniques for kicking, punching and throwing. In order to survive, you must improve yourself beyond your current abilities; physical, mental and spiritual. Becoming a black belt or master in some style of martial arts requires a new mindset and an evolution of your character that will take you to new heights in your art and in life.

A martial artist is concerned with many things in his training and in his life. He must learn all of the proper techniques for a given style of martial arts; he must consider studying other styles and weapons. He must develop powerful technique and good fighting ability and improve upon his character. There are thousands of training methods, drills, offenses and defenses. To become a black belt or a martial artist with a master's mindset you must seek excellence. ***Mediocrity is not acceptable.***

While there are many cookie-cutter martial arts schools that many of us like to call McDojos. They are willing to take your money and hand you a black belt in twelve to eighteen months along with a seriously false sense of accomplishment and self-confidence, a serious black belt can and should take years to earn and should not be rushed. Earning a black belt is a process of maturing in technique, strategy and character. Once you have climbed the mountain called black belt, you are ready for anything.

## *Commitment*

Black belts are just ordinary people, but with extraordinary commitment and that's what sets them apart. You will never achieve success in anything until you are committed to it. I can't tell you how many people walked through United Karate's doors and expressed great interest in martial arts. They would not think twice about spending a lot of time describing their fascination and admiration of martial arts and those who study them. That is where their involvement in martial arts ended. They stopped in essentially to tell us that they were interested admirers.

Other visitors simply walked in and said, "Where do I sign?" So what's the difference? Simple, one was interested and the other was committed. Now do you see? Our society is full of dreamers and doers, and a rare, lucky few are blessed to have both qualities. Dreaming and doing ultimately lead to success; whether it's earning your black belt, climbing the corporate ladder or achieving some other meaningful and challenging personal goal. Commitment keeps you going when you begin to waiver. There will be slumps and setbacks, you will reach plateaus and maybe even a few brick walls, but persistence will eventually get you there. Commit to your own success and keep that commitment fresh and clear in your mind and you will travel far!

## More than a Black Belt; a Martial Artist

Earning a black belt is not the same as *becoming* a black belt or more specifically a martial artist. Someone seeking to earn a black belt should strive to achieve much more than simply earning rank in a system of martial techniques. If that is your highest goal, then you are missing the point entirely. When you earn a black belt, you have acquired a great power; the power to kill, injure, maim or *not* kill; and with great power comes great responsibility. I hope that simply *earning* a black belt is not the sum total of your martial arts goals, but that *being* a black belt is what you aspire to. There is a world of difference.

Traditional martial arts requires adherence to a code of conduct and character. In almost every society where warriors and martial artists of various types have existed throughout history, the Japanese Samurai, the Korean Hwa Rang warriors, the Knights of Europe and even modern military forces, there has been the expectation that these highly trained warriors be governed and constrained by a code of conduct. The Samurai called it Bushido – Warrior Way - which dictated everything from social graces to etiquette on the battlefield. Warriors are expected to be servants of society and people of virtue as a means of balancing and controlling their lethal capabilities. In today's society, these same virtues and qualities are still admired, valued and sought after by us and for our children who are studying martial arts.

The goal for you or your child is to develop tools, techniques and qualities that are ready to translate into any aspect of life, wherever life may take you. Using martial arts character qualities in every aspect of your life can bring countless rewards and improve the quality of your life.

## *Achievement: A Personal Story*

Children and adults need focus, routine, structure, prioritization of goals and balance in their lives so that they can focus on fewer goals that they may actually achieve and gain that sense of confidence and accomplishment they seek. That is a path toward greater happiness. Martial arts are a proven way to develop these skills. Think long-term, but act short-term.

If you let small things get in your way, you will easily loose sight of your goals. The thing that is different about a martial artist is how he or she puts setbacks in perspective. To put them in the proper perspective, you must first recognize them for what they are. A setback is temporary. It is not a defeat or failure unless you make it one by allowing it to prevent you from achieving your goal. It is temporary, not permanent. If your state of mind is such that a setback is a permanent obstruction between you and your purpose or goals, then the setback has become a failure. Remember Henry Ford's words. "If you think you can't, you're right." That is one time you don't want to be right.

I had been training for four years and was an advanced brown belt. I had learned the curriculum, practiced, and trained diligently. I was nearing the point when I would be ready to test for my novice black belt; the rank before first-degree black belt. One day at my apartment, I severed a nerve and two tendons in the palm of my right hand on a piece of broken pottery. The injury required the efforts of a hand surgeon who stitched the nerve back together and repaired the tendons. I spent the next year going through intensive physical therapy just to regain the use of my hand. It was painful and certainly not fun.

During that time, I could not practice martial arts. I simply had to wait. I had to become healthy again and allow the injury to heal completely. During the year that I was out, the school changed their curriculum and I was told that I would not be able to finish what I had started and test under the old curriculum. I could keep my advanced brown-belt rank, but would have to learn the entire new curriculum from white belt.

Here I was so close to being ready for novice black belt only to find that I had to start all over again. All of my work and progress had been completely wiped out – or had it? I accepted that setback, recognizing it for what it was – a temporary event. I had made a commitment to myself when I started martial arts that I *was* going to achieve black belt. That was the goal I had set and I was not going to let that change of curriculum deter me. I began learning the new curriculum. After a year of no training or physical activity, I had to begin my conditioning again.

I used the four years of martial arts training that I had to that point to help me learn the new curriculum and become better than I had been at the old curriculum. The additional time allowed me to improve my technique and other skills. I was not really starting from scratch. I dived in, worked through the curriculum until I was ready for my novice black belt test. I passed that test with high marks and went on eighteen months later to pass my first-degree black belt test.

I had been an advanced brown belt for four years; a rather long time. The way I saw it, I was marinating. I wanted to be well-seasoned when I finally did become a black belt. All together, it took eight long years to earn my first-degree black belt. It seemed like forever. The wait was well worth it. The accomplishment was that much sweeter and I proved to myself that I could stick with a goal and not be deterred.

In my office, I have a picture frame on the wall that is a reminder to me about the value and importance of focus, perseverance and determination. The certificate in that frame, like my first-degree black belt, took much longer to earn than I would have hoped, but the experience was another object lesson in determination. Like the quest to complete my first-degree black belt, the experience changed my life. The frame contains my Bachelor's degree.

Many people have Bachelor's degrees and not many of them are worth much unfortunately, because people do not always use them to reach their potential. They are often merely a ticket to a job, not a stepping-stone in a personal journey. To me, my degree is different. I earned it twenty-four years after I began it. There were many points along the way where I had to stop for various reasons; some by choice and some not. The dream and the desire never left me nor did the determination. The result was that I completed that academic marathon and it has made a huge difference in my life and career.

Earning my black belt actually gave me the added confidence and determination to continue working through and complete my Bachelor's degree. It has brought opportunities and helped me develop more character along the way. It was not always easy, but nothing really worth doing ever is. This is success; but you must recognize your successes so that you can build upon them. The attainment of my degree was not the real measure of success. The success was the change in me and the character and perseverance that I developed to complete that quest. Since that time I went on with my wife (also a black belt) and three other instructors and we founded the very successful United Karate Institute of Self Defense, Inc., which we ran for many years. Anything is possible.

**Dream | Commit | Achieve**

## *Setting and Achieving Goals*

Martial arts learning and growth begins *again* at black belt. Unfortunately, many students don't realize that it is important to set higher goals long before reaching their black belt.

Do not lose sight of your goal. There are many small victories you can achieve along the way. Celebrate them. Look at setbacks as opportunities for victories not defeats. Those are the real accomplishments. You must consider that what you gain and the character that you develop from overcoming setbacks along the way to your goal is actually more valuable than obtaining the goal itself.

For some, these goals are personal. They might include a comprehensive knowledge of self-defense. For others, who have dedicated themselves to continue on after their black belt level is achieved; the goals might be a second or third degree. For still other individuals, personal development after black belt goes far beyond maintenance of physical skills or rank.

These individuals may wish to study other styles to improve their ability to defend themselves and others. Or perhaps it is a classical weapon, or the ability to excel at power techniques like breaking that becomes their goal. Other martial artists wish to test their skills in sport karate tournaments. Expression of their competitive spirit can be found in forms, fighting, and weapons. And finally, there are a few who wish to achieve their goals through the development of leadership and personal excellence. For these individuals, reaching their personal best is a lifetime goal. That is the primary theme of my book, ***"The Way of the Martial Artist: Achieving Success in Martial Arts and in Life!"*** Chapter 5 is titled, "Success for Life" and provides an important definition of success with 17 key steps toward achieving goals and a discussion of the five elements of success.

Whether a student wishes to pursue an advanced degree or to pursue another style, many options exist for those very few committed and dedicated students who progress beyond their initial black belt rank.

Why do we do the things that we do? The simple, answer is that almost everything that we do on a daily basis is part of accomplishing some goal, whether we consciously think about the goals or not. When we are hungry we eat. Eating accomplishes the goal of removing our hunger. When we are tired, we sleep or rest to satisfy the need for sleep. There are many short-term and long-term goals that we accomplish or set for ourselves. In martial arts and self defense we also have goals.

Goals in martial arts may be concerned with earning our next belt or earning our next achievement stripe on our current belt. We may be concerned about gaining more flexibility in our legs to kick a little higher or a little faster. There are hundreds of small and large goals that we can and should set for ourselves in martial arts. These goals give us a sense of purpose and when we accomplish them we experience a little boost in our self confidence and our self esteem. Every goal is a stepping stone to the next. ***Each goal that we accomplish makes us that much better prepared to set new goals and to take on new challenges.***

Whenever you are setting goals for yourself there are several important steps that you should take to help get you to your goals.

1. **Write down your goals.** When people write down their goals, the goals somehow take on a life of their own. When a goal is only talked about or thought of, and not actually written down, it doesn't seem very realistic or important. Once you write down your goals you are committing yourself to accomplishing them.

2. **Be specific.** Don't just write down that you want to get higher kicks. Write down that you are going to kick six inches higher in six months and six inches higher in another six months on your round kick. On your side kick, you are going to kick four inches higher in six months and so on.

   Don't just say that you are going to get your black belt. Say that you are going to get your black belt in three years and six months. Then figure out how many months that gives you at each belt level so that you can stay on schedule to test for your black belt.

3. **Write down the reasons why** you want to accomplish each of these goals? You may decide that some goals are not as important and others are more important. Writing the reasons down helps you see where you are coming from and where you are going.

4. **Make a list of resources.** Break your goal down into sub-goals until you can clearly see everything you must do to meet the main goal. Once you have done that, make a list of things that you will need to do each of these sub-goals. These are your resources.

   Your list of resources may include things like time - "I need twenty minutes per day to stretch and become more flexible", - or "I need to get some running shoes to start running regularly to increase my aerobic stamina." Figure out what you must have to accomplish your goals and get these items so that you will have what you need to get started.

5. **Make a schedule**. Look at your goals. You may be working on more than one goal at a time. Be careful not to take on too much at once. Be realistic. If you think that you have too many goals and not enough time or other resources, then pick the three most important goals and focus on them for now.

6. **Look at your schedule on a daily, weekly or monthly basis** and figure out how these goals fit. Draw up a chart or table with the items in your schedule and your new goals and follow you schedule. You may find that some adjustments to your schedule are necessary as you begin. Juggle some items around until you feel comfortable with the order of your activities. Don't sacrifice too much of your free time or sleep just to meet your goals. Free time for fun and relaxation is your reward for working hard and being consistent.

7. **Keep a log book**. Invest in a simple notebook or spiral notebook or daily/weekly planner. Find something that allows

you to keep track of your goals and your schedule. Use this log book daily to check off what you have accomplished. By writing down your progress and accomplishments, you will see and feel the progress you have made. The goals will seem more real and the progress will too!

8. **Evaluate your progress**. Once in a while, look at your logbook and determine if you are on track towards your goals. If you are not, then there are two likely reasons. One is that you are not sticking to your schedule. The other is that your schedule may not be very realistic.

   If you decided to become a black belt in three months and you are a white belt, chances are you won't make it! Each belt level requires a minimum of 30 lessons at many schools. There can be as many as eleven belt levels to reach 1st degree black belt. That's 330 lessons in six months. That means that you would have to go seven days per week, 4 times per day! No one can take that many lessons and test for a new belt once per month!

9. **Assess your schedule** and make sure that your goal is doable in the time frame that you are considering. It's perfectly ok to say, "Hey I think this goal is going to take longer than I thought. Now I'm going to adjust my deadlines and schedule to make it more attainable."

10. **Post your goals.** Find a good place at home or work to post your goals on a single sheet of paper. Make them clear and bold. Put them in order of priority or importance. At the bottom of the sheet sign your name. By signing your name, you are making a contract with yourself and committing yourself to stick to it. Every time that you see your goals, you will be reminded of what you have to do. Below is an example of how you can post your goals:

I, John Doe, hereby commit myself to accomplish the following personal goals. I am serious and determined to accomplish these goals to improve my martial arts skill and knowledge and my own value to myself.

1. Read one martial arts book every 6 weeks.
2. Stretch for 10 minutes each morning and 20 minutes each evening.
3. Run 3 miles, 3 times per week.
4. Compete in three tournaments per year.
5. Earn a new belt every three months.

5/21/2011
John H. Doe

11. **Read your goals**. Read your goals at the beginning of the day and sometime just before you go to bed. You will be constantly reminded of them and they will always be in your thoughts. Successful people are not necessarily any smarter, richer or more talented than the rest of us. They simply keep their sights on their goals and don't let little things get in the way. Accomplishing goals means having a plan and these ten steps help you to develop your plan.

12. **Reward yourself**. Every time you reach a major stepping stone or accomplish a goal reward yourself. It doesn't matter how small the goal is, if you planned it out and accomplished it, then reward yourself. Buy yourself an ice cream cone, a new album or a new dress or jacket or take one afternoon off from everything else and do something that you really enjoy. If you have stuck to your plan and completed something, that is worth celebrating! Tell others of your success also. These things will help build your self esteem and sense of accomplishment.

In the appendices I have included a goal worksheet that you can use to get started defining, understanding and organizing your goals. Review it, fill it out, post it and track your progress!

## Resources

**Books:**

1. The Way of the Martial Artist: Achieving Success in Martial Arts and in Life! – Kevin Brett
2. Warrior Wisdom: Ageless Wisdom for the Modern Warrior – Dr. Bohdi Sanders
3. The Book of Five Rings – Miyamoto Musashi (The Greatest Japanese Swordsman)
4. The Unfettered Mind: Writings of the Zen Master to the Sword Master – Takuan Soho
5. Bow to Life: 365 Secrets from the Martial Arts for Daily Life
6. Karate-Do: My Way of Life – Master Gichin Funakoshi (founder of Shotokan Karate)
7. The Karate Way: Discovering the Spirit of Practice – Dave Lowry
8. The Essence of Budo: A Practitioner's Guide to Understanding the Japanese Martial Ways – Dave Lowry

# Chapter 2

# *Transforming Our Children's Character through Martial Arts*

*"Martial arts should promote strength of character not merely physical technique. "*

## *Transformation for Life*

I like the line that the Marines use in their commercials, *"The transformation is for life."* Transformation is a big word and in short it means a big change. Something significant has changed for the better. We want those positive changes in our children. If we could wave a magic wand and sprinkle pixy dust on our little ones so that they possessed ample amounts of virtues and positive qualities our job as parents and instructors would be finished. Wake up, you're not in Kansas anymore, it isn't that simple.

The job of molding the character of our youth, the next generation of our society, is the responsibility and the privilege of dedicated parents, school teachers, mentors, and martial arts instructors. How exactly that is accomplished is not quite as simple as teaching kicking and punching. These martial arts virtues and values that you see advertised by every martial arts school as a stock advertising slogan are often overlooked or worse, not even addressed or emphasized throughout the development in many schools. I don't say that to be discouraging, but just to make you aware that that is one of the topics you want to discuss with potential schools and their instructors or owners. The real question is "What do you teach and how?" I have seen schools that are actual leadership academies where character building is the central theme that weaves its way through all of the training, advancement and requirements. They have a true academy approach to training.

In the corporate or government world it is commonplace when there are particular messages or points to be communicated to a given audience that someone drafts a communications plan. This plan is then the blueprint for teaching and educating the intended audience on these critical topics and messages. A training plan is often a close companion to the communications plan. A communications plan describes four things:

## Communications Plan

**Question 1:** Who is the audience?
**Answer:** *In this case your children*

**Question 2:** What messages do you want to convey?
**Answer:** *The values and virtues of martial arts*

**Question 3:** In what venues (locations or settings) will the message be conveyed?
**Answer:** *Dojo and at home*

**Question 4:** How will these messages be conveyed?
**Answer:** *Discussions with parents and instructors, stories that teach a point, instructors or parents leading by example to demonstrate the tenets or virtues, drills, workshops or specially designed exercises or scenarios that allow children to act out how they would apply a lesson, value or virtue in daily life. These messages can also be conveyed in situations where the child might use or benefit from various martial arts virtues such as respect, confidence, etc.*

So if we look at the questions in our communications plan for teaching and instilling martial arts virtues in our children, we can begin to see where there are many messages that can be conveyed in many contexts and situations and in many ways to help our children learn and understand these life-changing concepts.

There are some key elements to instilling the messages and values that we must keep in mind. These valuable lessons must be communicated often and in a variety of situations and settings so that our children can assimilate and internalize the messages and their application or significance to their life. Question four in the box above really gets at the idea of the training plan. If you have something that you want your children to be capable of understanding, internalizing and exhibiting as part of their normal behavior and character then they will need to be trained; immersed in it; exposed to it and rehearsed in it.

As you and your marital arts school begin to immerse your children in the positive, enriching and life-changing virtues and tenets of martial arts, you will be exposing them to positive and constructive ideas that can ultimately help them succeed in martial arts, in school, in relationships and as a member of your family and community. It is every parent's wish that as these values take hold and become a part of your child's makeup and abilities and that these learning experiences will carry forward with them into their adult lives and help provide meaning, purpose and direction on their future journeys.

Martial arts instructors have a training plan for the punching and kicking and the physical fitness aspects of preparing them for advancement to their next belt or rank level. The training plan is essentially the entire martial arts curriculum that is required for each belt level. What we're talking about in this chapter is the character component of your child's training that may not actually be a conscious part of the training plan at the martial arts school. Below are some simple ideas that you can discuss or hopefully your child's instructors will discuss with your children. The goal is to augment your child's martial arts training. You want to ensure that the character development aspects are emphasized in their training and translated into their daily life at home, school, church, playgrounds and elsewhere.

Review these and discuss with your children different ways that each of these virtues can be shown and accomplished in their daily life. It's easy to talk about them, but talk about how to actually make them work in real life so that next time your child is in a situation where one or more of these virtues might apply, they will have some ideas already in their head about what to do and you will also be able to provide some simple queue for them to remember your discussions and practice what they have learned. Talk while you are driving in the car, at the dinner table, while taking a walk or take a few minutes at night before you tuck them in to bed. Review the concept in different ways for many days in a row and then come back to it again a few weeks or months later. I hate to use the analogy, but it's like training a dog; just a few times won't do the trick. It will require continuous reinforcement over a long period of time until these values and character qualities become internalized, programmed in and automatic. Then you know you have done your job.

***"Look at how to make the next level of improvement from where you are. This is how excellence is achieved."***

## Patience

**Meaning:** Patience is accepting the situation and working with it for what it is without becoming upset, angry or frustrated.

**Messages**: When something or someone is a challenge, patience can allow you to deal with the situation more successfully to get better at something or relate better to someone and make you happy that you did so.

**Examples:**

- Patience to wait without interrupting while adults complete a conversation.
- Patience to practice a new martial arts technique, a math problem or other challenge for many repetitions or for an extended period of time in order to improve gradually without expecting instant mastery of something.
- Patience with another person who may be annoying or irritating
- Patience with yourself so that you don't get frustrated too easily and become upset or angry.

**How it's Relevant:**

Exercising patience can bring satisfaction by resulting in a better outcome than giving up in frustration. A challenge requires patience, but on the other side of that challenge can be rewarding accomplishment and achievement and improved self-esteem and self-confidence because your child persevered and did not give up. Giving up on something too quickly can damage self-esteem and self-confidence and only begins to instill an attitude of failure. When something is challenging or difficult, see it through to completion. That is an attitude for success!

## Determination and Perseverance

**Meaning:** Determination and perseverance are similar to patience, but I think of these as more aggressive while patience is passive acceptance of a situation. Determination is a more assertive act where your child is resolved and committed to continue on and push through to accomplish a task or achieve some level of performance in the short term or the long term.

**Messages**: Determination is a no-quitting attitude that helps you overcome challenges, get where you want to be or accomplish an immediate goal or a long-term goal that will require much effort. Determination every day and commitment to the goal will keep you going and get you closer to where you want to be.

### Examples:

- Determination to learn a new martial arts technique.
- Determination to keep pushing hard during a workout and use extra energy.
- Determination to work smart and work hard to study and prepare to learn the material for a test in school.
- Determination not to talk in class or be disruptive.

### How it's Relevant:

Simply trying harder or digging deep from inside to have the mental commitment and applying the physical energy to keep going can get you through a tiring activity, exercise or obstacle. Making progress toward a goal because you made a short-term or long-term commitment and were determined to achieve progress and stayed with it will make you more confident that you can overcome other obstacles and challenges.

## Respect

**Meaning:** The ability to appreciate the significance of what someone else has achieved or has to say. To appreciate someone else's rank, position, title, experience and hold it in high esteem without feeling that you are inferior.

**Messages:** Respecting someone else or someone else's property does not lessen what you are or have accomplished. It may be a way to recognize where you would like to be or simply that someone else in their experiences has achieved much and has developed the qualities required to achieve significant things. Look at this as an opportunity to learn from someone more accomplished and see what lessons might help you. Showing respect to others can help them respect you and treat you in a positive way as well.

### Examples:

- Respect for a teacher or instructor will lead to being able to pay closer attention and learn from them.
- Respect for someone who does not agree with you does not mean you are giving in or changing your opinion, but you can still appreciate that their opinion is important to them.
- Respect for someone else's property means taking care of it if you are allowed to use or borrow something of theirs. It also means not touching something that is not yours or which you have not been given permission to hold.

### How it's Relevant:

Respect can improve or maintain a relationship and how well you may relate to someone else and this can bring rewards of better relationships.

## Discipline

**Meaning:** Doing what you are told is exercising discipline. Following instructions and not pushing back or arguing about what is asked of you is following discipline.

**Messages:**
Discipline comes from the outside and when you follow orders or directions from someone else, you are showing them respect by complying. As you follow an instructor's direction, you are helping them teach you and you have an opportunity to learn and grow. Discipline is learning what is necessary and what must be done and beginning to develop useful habits, routines and patterns of behavior that are helpful and give structure to your life.

**Examples:**
- Discipline to do something difficult as someone pushes you to achieve more than you thought you might be able to accomplish.
- Discipline to comply and follow a pattern or expectation of action, conduct or behavior usually in the course of maintaining order for learning.

**How it's Relevant:**
Discipline is the first step toward establishing and growing into self-discipline. Discipline or being taught discipline means developing the ability to follow orders and directions which are essential for an orderly and civil society. As a student or child learns to respond positively to discipline, they are becoming more trustworthy and dependable and learning where the boundaries of acceptable behavior are and what consequences might result from stepping outside the bounds. These conditions actually can bring more reassuring feeling about what will be accepted or tolerated and what is not.

## Self-Discipline, Restraint & Tolerance

**Meaning:** Self-discipline means doing what is right without having to be told. Self-discipline is internally driven. You do what you know is right even when your parents, boss, instructor or other authority is not present. Restraint or self-restraint is closely related to self-discipline. It is holding back (out of respect) from saying or doing something you might regret. It is using good choices to maintain control over your anger or disagreement with someone or something.

### Messages:

Self-Discipline is doing what is necessary, beneficial or difficult even when you do not feel like it. Restraint is related to tolerance because restraint is sometimes needed to be tolerant of someone or something that you do not like or with whom you do not agree. Tolerance does not mean you must subject yourself to someone else's abuses however. If someone is being abusive in any way, that is where your self-esteem, and confidence should kick in to give you the courage to stand up to the abusive person and let them know that you will not tolerate their behavior. Martin Luther King Jr. said, "Let us not become so tolerant that we tolerate intolerance."

### Examples:

- When you practice extra math problems for homework or start your homework on your own without having to be told.
- When you show up early to martial arts class and practice kicks or kata on your own so that you can improve.
- Restraint is how you can keep from yelling at someone, being disrespectful or doing what you might want to say or do when you know it is wrong.
- Someone expressing an opinion with which you disagree is not necessarily being abusive. When someone is taking advantage of or treating others in a demeaning or negative way and using their opinion as an excuse, this is behavior that should not be tolerated.

### How it's Relevant:

Self-discipline can help you through challenges in school, work, home or wherever and parents, teachers and instructors appreciate self-discipline because it means that you will do what is needed without having to be told every time. That is helpful and shows maturity.

## Leadership

**Meaning:** Leadership is the ability to motivate and direct others to accomplish what you or they need to accomplish.

**Messages:** Leadership is taking charge directly or indirectly by motivating and exciting others toward a goal and through challenges and difficulties. There are many qualities to a good leader; leading by example; leading from behind, by motivating and providing the opportunity for others to lead and advance or accomplish goals. Leaders must provide and communicate a vision, goal or objective. They must educate or communicate to those whom they will lead what is important about the goal and why and motivate them to see the task through to completion. Leadership is most successful with positive motivation, but there are cases when stern, disciplined leadership is necessary to maintain drive and direction. Leaders often encourage others to excel where they did not think they could and to find and bring out the best in people. Leadership has many styles, but the most effective leaders must care about those they lead and listen to them as well.

### Examples:

- Leading; taking charge and responsibility for a family, leading a church group, leading a school group on a project, leading a military unit, a scouting unit, a project at work.
- Leading others to safety after a natural disaster.
- Children may lead others to safety and act as a source of encouragement and motivation in a dangerous school incident or shooting.

### How it's Relevant:

Life will provide many opportunities and necessary situations where you must exercise leadership. Successfully handling these situations on your own or with a group may depend upon your leadership abilities and qualities. Leadership can be rewarding, exciting and motivational to inspire you with more self-confidence to excel to greater height in life, work, family and relationships.

## Self-Confidence & Courage

**Meaning:** Self-Confidence is having the knowledge to know that something is possible because you have done that particular thing before or that something new is possible because you have accomplished other difficult challenges and are assured that you can find a way to achieve or accomplish this new thing. Courage is closely related to self-confidence. With self-confidence, courage is possible. Courage is not the lack of fear, but the willingness to do something in spite of fear that you might have.

**Messages:** Confident people may still be uncertain, scared or unsure of themselves at times, but that is where the self-confidence kicks in and helps them over that hump and onward to take on new challenges. It is the knowledge that somehow, inside you is the ability to do something or at least to find a way to do it. It is an internal drive where you urge yourself on with determination and perseverance to break new ground and try new things even if there is a risk of failure; understanding that failure is only failure when you do not grow or learn something from the experience.

**Examples:**

- Standing up to peer pressure or bullies and refusing to give in to their demands, dares or insults.
- Trying new activities and experiences which will result in growth and even stronger confidence.
- Courage is useful if you have to stand up to a bully or an assailant in a self-defense situation.
- Courage is what it takes to admit you made a mistake or did something wrong.

**How it's Relevant:**

Self-confidence is much like courage. Even when you may not be certain of the outcome, you are willing to try. And when there is something that you definitely know how to do, you have no doubt that you can accomplish what you need and when you need it. Self-confidence helps overcome initial fears and concerns with willingness and bravery. Without a strong self-confidence and determination, many fun, rewarding and important experiences and accomplishments in life may never be realized.

## Self-Respect/Self-Esteem

**Meaning:** Self-respect or self-esteem means having a healthy, positive opinion of yourself as a person and your own sense of self-worth. In other words, you are important just because you are you. This is not egotistical, but just a strong sense that you are worthy of being treated well and should not be subject to abusive, degrading or demeaning treatment.

**Messages:** Self-esteem or having a strong sense of self-respect means you will not tolerate being treated badly and that you should not be subject to negative or disrespectful or emotionally damaging behavior.

### Examples:

- A parent, teacher, instructor, boyfriend, girlfriend, husband, wife or child cannot and should not treat you disrespectfully or badly. You do not deserve that type of treatment. No one is perfect, but mistakes or errors in judgment do not mean that you deserve to be treated poorly in any situation.
- Self-esteem is related to self-confidence. As you develop more confidence in your abilities to do things, you should think about that - reflect on it. You are growing, becoming better and that is something to be proud of.
- You can help build and maintain someone's self-esteem by complementing them when they do a good job on something. That can make them feel better about themselves and their abilities.

### How it's Relevant:

Self-esteem combined with self-confidence is an important part of growing, maturing and reaching outward and upward to new heights and new experiences. Someone who is low in self-esteem and has little self-respect will allow others to treat them however they may feel and may even feel like they deserve the poor treatment. This is completely false! You must work to improve your self-esteem and self-respect by taking even small steps toward new achievements and new experiences that can be rewarding, fulfilling and confidence-building.

## Goal-Setting and Achieving Excellence

**(Planning & Organization)**

**Meaning:** Think big, be aggressive, reach far, and strive for high goals.

**Messages:** Setting goals and working toward them provides rewarding and enriching experiences, develops new skills and builds confidence. There is usually a reason for setting and attempting a goal. Understand this reason. It will help you prepare better and to better understand what is motivating you. Learn about what it takes to set goals, prepare for the challenges that will be involved, develop a positive mindset and outlook on approaching challenges and organizing your life around accomplishing excellence in everything you do. There is an old saying that there is only a one degree temperature difference between when water boils and when it is just hot water. That one degree of extra effort, planning or work could be the difference between being ok at something and being excellent!

### Examples:

- Setting a goal to become a 1st degree black belt and practicing diligently to improve your techniques and your knowledge to become an excellent skilled and well-educated black belt.
- Rather than seek perfection, seek continuing excellence and improvement. Don't look at what is not attainable (perfection), look at how to make the next level of improvement from where you are. This is how excellence is achieved. Look at how to accomplish the next task that will bring you closer to your goal.

### How it's Relevant:

You will not always achieve high goals or maybe not in the time you might like. When you reach and fall short, you are still building your character and learning where your abilities may fall short of what is required to accomplish a goal. If you do not achieve a goal, that is not failure, but a lesson in what you may need to accomplish first (needed skills, resources or planning) before you might actually achieve the goal.

## Physical Fitness
**(Nutrition & Healthy Living)**

**Meaning:** Physical fitness is maintaining a physically active life-style to keep energy levels high and to maintain good health so that you feel good. This requires learning about good eating habits, training habits and ensuring plenty of sleep; avoiding junk and learning what a healthy diet is and getting in good amounts of exercise to build strength, endurance and flexibility.

**Messages:** A healthy life-style makes life more exciting and enjoyable. People with healthy life-styles live longer, are happier and feel better more of the time than those without. Don't be over committed or over active at least without equal amounts of nothingness - inactivity - downtime. Balance will require time to mentally and physically decompress after much physical or mental activity.

### Examples:

- Avoiding too many sodas, sweets, ice cream and other high calorie foods and eating more fruit, veggies, fiber, fish, and poultry!
- Being active daily with some physical activity and balancing that with adequate rest.

### How it's Relevant:

Too many Americans are coming down with diabetes at very young ages solely due to terrible diets. Many health problems are associated with diabetes and can be completely prevented with healthy food and exercise instead of fast food and large amounts of processed foods. Avoid serious health problems by developing good eating and exercise habits young so they will carry with you into adulthood. Too many people and their children are involved in too many activities at any one time. Few of them have the time to achieve excellence or to have a quality experience in the activities they are involved in. They are merely chasing after mediocrity - less is more. Seek quality, not quantity and balance in all things.

# Life Skills

**(Listening skills, conflict resolution, anger management)**

**Meaning:** Listening is taking in someone else's message, thought, feelings or argument. Conflict resolution is trying to solve an issue without feeling the need to win or to surrender; to balance. Anger management is approaching a situation with a perspective that is different than your usual viewpoint that would cause you anger.

**Messages:** Too many of us hear, but we do not listen. If we would stop, focus and target our mental energy only on the thoughts of what a person is telling or teaching us or warning us about, we could understand better what they are saying or feeling. To listen, we must empty our cup, open our mind, tune our senses and look at the person, hear the words and take them in. Clouding another person's message with too many of our own thoughts can cause misunderstandings. Many conflicts could be avoided if we would listen. Conflict resolution is seeking a solution without surrendering; hearing another's position, without abandoning yours; truly working to find a solution that is workable, not appeasing in the pursuit of peace.

## Examples:

- A disagreement; do not let your first interpretation of a situation lead you to anger. Change your perspective and you will change the outcome. If you see a situation in a different light, then you may gain new insights into why it happened or how to handle it other than becoming angry.
- Ask yourself why you are angry and what it would take to not be angry. What would need to be different? Maybe the person or the situation can't change, but the way you handle it or see it could.
- When you are asked to do a chore, think about the opportunity to make your parent happy and pleased that you are willing to do something for them and help out. It is different than being angry or creating a conflict about having to perform the chore. Make it positive and it will be positive.

## How it's Relevant:

Anger often happens because you always look at a situation that could anger you from the same perspective. If you apply better listening skills to pick up on what your boss, parents or coaches are saying you might not become angry, but rather more thankful that they are trying to help you and guide you.

## Focus & Concentration

(paying attention to small things that matter)

**Meaning:** Being able to stick with a task undistracted and determined to work through the details of it without letting up.

### Messages:

Practicing focus and concentration drills will help strengthen your ability to concentrate. This could become a life-saving skill. Being too easily distracted could have serious consequences in different situations.

### Examples:

- Practicing a kata while others are circled around you making distracting comments and laughing. Being able to perform the kata well with distractions requires and builds focus and concentration.
- Practice tasks like homework or reading with small distractions like having music on nearby or whatever might be considered a distraction, simply to quiet the mind and tune out your surroundings so that you might only see and hear what you are reading or writing.
- Think of various practice drills in martial arts or even in conducting a conversation with someone. You are trying to concentrate on what they are saying in the midst of several distractions like the television.

### How it's Relevant:

Focus and concentration are critical in school, work, relationships and life. Focus and concentration are skills that take practice and yet as you improve at them you will be able to be more productive and have more positive experiences rather than confusion because you have not been able to focus well enough to take in the situation or see what is right in front of you.

## Responsibility

**Meaning:** Responsibility is having the courage and confidence to stand up and take ownership. Responsibility really means that you recognize your involvement in a situation and that you must become the owner of that situation by taking responsibility. If something has not gone as planned, leadership demands that the responsible party accept the consequences and deal with them rather than avoid consequences or pass the blame to someone else.

**Messages**:
When you take responsibility for something, good or bad, you are acknowledging to yourself or others that it is up to you and not someone else to take action and correct a potentially wrong situation.

**Examples:**
If you damage something you borrowed from someone else you must fix or replace it. Even if you borrowed something and a friend or relative caused the damage, you must take responsibility because the item was under your control and you were in charge of safeguarding the item until it was returned to its owner.

**How it's Relevant:**
Responsibility is a leadership quality. Taking responsibility for accomplishing a task, a mission, an objective or some project means you are assuming the lead and others will look to you for direction. This is a chance to grow, to build your own confidence and to instill confidence in others about your abilities. If you demonstrate that you will follow through on your responsibilities this can translate into future opportunities and you will develop a reputation as someone who can be counted upon.

## Kindness & Service

**Meaning:** A martial artist is a type of warrior. The idea comes from Asian traditions such as the Japanese Samurai which means "one who serves". Kindness is the willingness to help others, to show compassion and care for those who may be broken or hurting physically or emotionally. Service is what a martial artist does when he or she helps others out in different ways or serves his family, community, school, military unit or other group. Kindness is a sign of confidence, assuredness and strength.

**Messages:** There is an ancient concept used in Asia and Medieval Europe with many of the warrior traditions and knighthood where the warriors are expected to put service to others above self. A martial artist should find and serve a purpose outside of him or herself and give back to society by trying to improve the conditions or circumstances of those around or dependent upon him. By doing so, these are acts of service and kindness. The first hospitals were created to care for the sick and injured by warriors called the Knights Hospitallers. Many other acts of compassion and kindness have been rendered by other warrior cultures and organizations. Of those to whom much skill, power and lethality has been given or entrusted, much service and support is expected.

**Examples:**

- Aiding others in an emergency.
- Assisting or protecting someone younger or weaker than you from being bullied.
- Helping a lower ranking student or a sibling with their homework.
- Helping a co-worker with accomplishing a challenging assignment.
- Be honest and up-front with someone who needs to hear the hard truth about something instead of telling them what they want to hear.

**How it's Relevant:** A civilized society without kindness and service – is not civilized. How could it be any more relevant?

Certainly there is much more that could be said about any of these topics. The best I can do in these few short pages is to bring the topics to your attention and give you some guidelines for how to view them and engage with your instructors and children to work through illuminating your children about these positive concepts. One further idea that may be useful is to pick a virtue for the month as many public school systems do and work through many examples, stories, situations and potential play-acting scenarios where these lessons can be applied. Most important though is consistency and keeping the positive messages and lessons coming so that they begin to creep into their conscious and sub-conscious. Eventually these values will take hold as your children begin to internalize them and make them part of who they are and how they act. I close this chapter with a couple of illustrative stories that I think provide good lessons and food for thought for you parents.

## *Programming in Humility and a Dose of Respect*

At United Karate, we had a family where the father was a black belt and he had a nine-year old daughter and an eight year old son who were both black belts. The kids were good kids and they had transferred over to our school from another when we opened. While they had received their black belts in a fairly short period of time (18 to 22 months approximately) They were fairly competent technically. The boy, however, was having some disrespect issues and was not showing even a reasonable degree of respect toward the instructors. He was disruptive in class and often bragged significantly about how much better he was than others and was often demeaning toward lower ranking students rather than being helpful toward them. In short, he was not acting like a martial artist. He had simply earned a rank. His father was not pleased with his behavior and attitude either and his grades in school had taken a nosedive about the same time the attitude began to set in. Granted, we're talking about a young boy here, not an adult, but that's where the attitudes begin.

When an under belt student (someone below the rank of black belt) is disrespectful or disruptive in class he or she is given a warning. The second time we have them sit out for fifteen minutes of the class. The third time they are disruptive or if they even show blatant disrespect inside or outside of class, we ask them to take off their belt and hand it to us. We then hang the belt on the balance bar and tie it in place where it is a visible reminder that we gave the rank and we can remove it when they act in a manner that is unbecoming of a martial artist.

With this young black belt, we had noticed this problem over many classes. With a black belt, however, you generally do not take or touch their belt. This was a special case. One day during class, he was being disrespectful *again*. I calmly asked him to come forward. He walked up to the front of class as the others stood at attention. I continued in a calm tone and asked him to remove his belt. He went pale; looked down at his belt, realizing this was serious. He removed his belt and handed it to me. It was the first time we had removed a black belt and tied it on the bar. I told him that he was to attend white-belt through red-belt classes for one month. He was not allowed to attend any brown and black belt classes during this time. I also announced that after a month of under belt review he would have an opportunity to *earn* his belt back by performing the entire curriculum over again in front of the black belt class as an informal test before his peers. I also informed him that he was to write a paper of however many words he thought were appropriate explaining to me what it means to be a black belt.

The month passed. He attended classes with no belt. He had to swallow some pride and accept his circumstances and the consequences of his behavior that led him there. Once he had completed thirty lessons at the under belt level it was time to run him through his paces. He went through the entire curriculum and performed everything over again as if he were testing for black belt for the first time. He turned in his short essay and the other instructors and I reviewed the essay and briefly discussed his performance during the test. Once we had finished our mini conclave, we called him forward and presented him his belt and congratulated him. He had learned a valuable lesson in respect and humility and from that day forward, he became a model black belt, an outstanding student in school and was always seen eagerly helping younger students and putting in extra time teaching. He later went on as he became older and did very well in school. These are the kinds of life-changing events and lessons that happen every week in a good martial arts school.

## *Building Self-Esteem through Focus and Commitment*

There is a season for everything. We don't have to become schizophrenic and try to do everything at the same time. Apply the discipline to remain focused and you will see results and achieve happiness.

Today, parents feel that good parenting means signing up each child for several sports and activities in and out of school simultaneously. The reality is that somewhere in the mix, homework looses priority and children and parents become stressed. I have seen too many instances where a parent has to whisk their child away from a soccer game before it is over, to take them to a baseball game. Other times, on many occasions, I have seen a parent take a child to a two-night scout campout beginning on a Friday night. The next morning, they leave before breakfast to go to a basketball game. They return to camp around lunchtime to participate for an hour or so in the camp activities, only to leave again in the mid-afternoon to go to a football game. Then they return after dinner to hang around the campfire, listening like some outsider to the other campers talk about the fun events of the day. What is my point? Well, if it is not already clear, the child does not complete any event or activity. Where is the sense of pride in accomplishment in that? The child cannot really feel like he or she is part of any of the groups because there are too many conflicting and overlapping activities. The child develops little of their potential because they simply do not have the time to become good at anything and actually enjoy it. Their parents are merely helping the child check a box and frankly the parents are being selfish because it is often their own guilt thinking that they must give their child everything; every opportunity. Certainly we want our children to have opportunities, but that does not mean we have to give them these opportunities all at the same time! Give them time to focus and excel.

The smart approach would be to limit the activities to one sport and one other activity per season. Over time, the child will still be able to participate in a variety of activities or sports, just not all at once! It seems obvious, but I have friends who have been doing this insane multi-taking for years and keep talking about how difficult and stressful it is. I have seen children at very young ages talk about how overwhelmed they are; sounding like some over-worked government employee who is being overloaded by trying to do the work of three or four people. I tell the parents to just stop, but they don't seem to feel that they have it within their power to run their own lives. Instead, they let their lives run them. A little focus with some prioritization will make life more balanced and enjoyable. Children and adults need this balance so that they can focus on fewer goals that they may actually achieve. Then as these goals are achieved and they gain skill and prowess they will develop the sense of confidence and accomplishment we all seek. That is a path toward greater happiness, high-achievement and success. With so much activity, there is no time for inactivity; peace and calmness. Too many people have lost the critical ability to do nothing.

## A Life-Changing Lesson in Perseverance and Achievement

Before we founded United Karate, my wife and other instructors were at a different martial arts school. We attended a black belt test where four of the candidates who were testing for their novice black belts were children. All four were age ten. They had been training several years to reach advanced brown belt. Unfortunately, they were not prepared for their novice black belt test and the instructor who pre-tested them should never have let them pass their pre-test.

Nonetheless, they were all deemed ready for their novice black belt test. The day of the test came, and after the adults had been tested on their kata, technical kicks, self-defense and knowledge questions, it was time for the children. The group of four came up and formed a line in front of the panel of judges. They were given the commands and put through their paces to demonstrate their curriculum. They were tested and quizzed on a variety of knowledge questions that all black belt candidates were required to know.

When the testing was completed, the chief instructors and the master of the school did not pass the four young candidates. They were told they could come back in six months and test again. Immediately after the test ended, the parents of two of the children were outraged. They expected their children to pass and literally assumed that paying of the testing fee and passing the pre-test virtually guaranteed passing; not so.

Those parents and their children left the school and their children never continued in martial arts. What a negative, defeatist attitude these parents instilled in their children. What do you think will happen the next time those children attempt something difficult or challenging and do not succeed the first time? It's probably a safe bet that they will simply give up and try something else. Enough of those kinds of experiences and they will learn that maybe they should not try to achieve any goals that might not work out perfectly the first time, so why bother at all?

The other two students met afterward with their parents. They were understandably surprised and disappointed after having passed their pre-test, but the beautiful part of this story is that those other two students showed true martial arts spirit. They were encouraged by their parents and for the next six months, they applied themselves diligently to learning what they had done wrong on the test and what they must do to improve.

They changed the way they practiced, prepared, and trained. They focused intently on their goal. They became more determined than ever. However, what they were determined about was not so much earning their black belt, but changing their ways. In that one instant, when they learned that they had failed their test, they did not see that as a failure as had the other children. These two young warriors saw that they had not prepared appropriately and realized that they needed to change their training routine.

The six months passed quickly. I watched the two students apply themselves in a serious, dedicated manner that an adult would be proud to exhibit. When the day of the test came, their techniques were a joy to watch. Their demonstration of the required knowledge portions of the test was impeccable. Their attitudes were upbeat, enthusiastic, determined and confident. They passed with outstanding scores.

A year later, they went on and passed their test for first-degree black belts in the same manner. They became student instructors, helping the adult instructors, assisting and teaching other children. They entered many tournaments, did very well and excelled in school. They were successful, not because they earned a black belt, but because they improved their character and attitude. This change led to a long string of successful outcomes in every aspect of their life.

The moral of the story? The challenges with which we are confronted provide us with an opportunity to shape our character. How will you shape yours?

# Resources

**Books:**

1. The Way of the Martial Artist: Achieving Success in Martial Arts and in Life! – Kevin Brett
2. Warrior Wisdom: The Heart and Soul of Bushido – Dr. Bohdi Sanders
3. Living the Martial Way : A Manual for the Way a Modern Warrior Should Think – Forest Morgan
4. The Peaceful Way: A Children's Guide to the Traditions of the Martial Arts – Claudio Iedwab, Roxane Standefer
5. Respect: Martial Arts Code Of Conduct - Terrence Webster-Doyle
6. My First Martial Arts Book (Martial Arts for Peace Series) – Terrence Webster-Doyle

# Chapter 3
# Self-Defense and Combat

*"The more realistic your training. The less shocking reality will be."*

## The Practical Need for Self-Defense

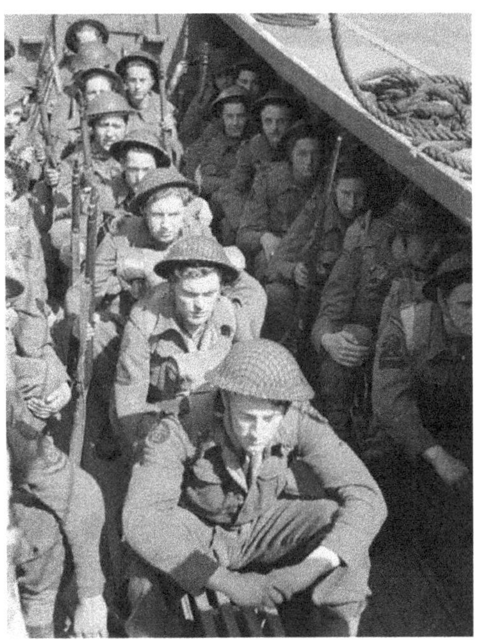

In the early days of World War II, England was in a desperate struggle for survival. The British Ministry of Defence was racing to equip its armed forces defensively to thwart a Nazi invasion of England. They prepared to stand up resistance efforts and to "set Europe ablaze" as Churchill ordered his British commando units. As England's outlook became bleaker, the Allied Forces gathered the worlds' leading combat experts. The day after Pearl Harbor was attacked, these experts met at a Top-Secret base "Camp-X" in Canada. Not even the Prime Minister of Canada knew of this facility's existence. The Allies began to create a secret weapon of mass destruction to defeat the Nazis.

Each G.I. and Marine carried this weapon with him. This weapon was truly an ancient Oriental secret. It was a set of highly lethal combative techniques distilled through years of successful use and refinement. These techniques were a veritable sampler platter taken from a broad cross-section of Asian martial arts. This dirty little secret was a training regime of easily learnable, virtually fool-proof techniques that transformed regular troops into a lethal force with just a few weeks of training. This power force struck fear in the heart of the Nazis.

In the years following Viet Nam, this type of training and these techniques fell into disuse; largely considered too lethal for less conventional military engagements and police actions. Today's military has adopted a more balanced approach to close-quarters combat to give our troops training and options to use non-lethal or lethal force. Today, as violent crimes and gangs spread across our society, regular citizens require a similar mixture of lethal and non-lethal self-defense techniques that can be learned quickly and easily without spending years studying martial arts.

Each branch of the military has its own varieties of hand-to-hand combat. These are simple techniques taught to provide our troops with basic skills for those situations where using a firearm is not a good choice or where they may have lost or damaged their weapon or run out of ammunition. The U.S. Marine Corps has even gone so far as to develop an entire full-fledged martial art of its own. This is known as the Marine Corps Martial Arts Program (MCMAP). All Marines are taught this system and required to earn at least the third belt (green) in the belt ranking system. There are no traditional forms or kata. The techniques are a combination of many useful hand-to-hand combat techniques derived from nearly 100 years of close-quarters combat development stretching back to the 1920s.

These techniques are generally known as combatives and generally are extremely simple and reliable, turning previously untrained soldiers and Marines into lethal weapons in a matter of a days or weeks. The genesis of much of this type of training was documented in the book, "Kill or Get Killed" by Colonel William Fairbairn (British Royal Marines) and eventually evolved over the years into training in the U.S. military and law enforcement.

My point in this brief history is that effective and lethal self-defense training need not take the many years it can take to earn a black belt and in fact, in most instances will be more effective than typical commercial black belt training which puts much emphasis on sport competition and simply learning the forms, patterns or kata as set routine with little if any practical and proven self-defense application of the techniques being taught.

Many of the techniques taught in self-defense classes can cause serious injury or even death to an assailant, so it is crucial to have only serious, mature students. This training is ideal for a wide range of individuals who would readily benefit from acquiring basic self-defense skills. These skills will help students develop confidence and competence in threatening situations.

Violence in our schools is increasing at an alarming rate. High school and college students simply must be capable of defending themselves. Young mothers, young men, and even middle-aged and older individuals are all potential beneficiaries of this type of training because no one is immune to threatening situations.

Truly effective self defense techniques require minimal strength and capitalize on the application of leverage and knowledge of vital areas. This makes these techniques ideal for many individuals, especially women who typically have less upper body strength than men.

The most effective self defense techniques are simple to execute and easy to learn. In a real self defense situation there is no time for complex techniques or motion picture style theatrics. The objective is simply to use the least force needed to allow the student to free themselves from the threat and escape from the scene of an assault.

*"There's no fair play; no rules except one: kill or get killed."*

Colonel William Fairbairn (British Royal Marines)
Father of Close-Quarters Combat: Author of "Kill or Get Killed"

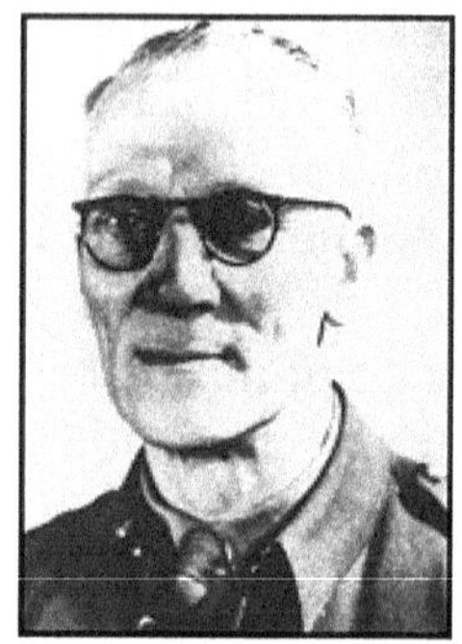

## *Modern Self-Defense Training*

I hope for your own safety that you are not one of those incredibly naïve folks who think you are big enough and strong enough to defend yourself and that's all you need or that you don't hang out in bad, dangerous areas, so you don't have anything to worry about. Those are exactly the types of people who need self-defense training the most. They are living under some seriously flawed assumptions and they don't even suspect that they are at risk. That very attitude puts them more at risk because they refuse to believe they are in any danger. Nothing could be further from the truth. Quit burying your head in the sand like an Ostrich and look around you. A violent assault is committed somewhere in the United States every seven seconds. That's a lot of victims, or as I prefer to view it, a lot of potential survivors.

You do not have to be a black belt to be able to defend yourself. Many people have the misconception that in order to adequately defend themselves they must be built like Arnold Schwartzeneger or that they must be some world class black belt capable of breaking a dozen bricks with their forehead. Nothing could be further from the truth. Below are a few basic tenets of self-defense that are vital to your survival.

## What is Self-Defense?

1. Self-defense is any technique, tactic or strategy that can be used to neutralize an assailant and escape.
2. Self-defense can employ defensive use of anything from hand-to-hand combat, clawing, scratching, biting, spitting, using pepper spray, knives, everyday objects used as makeshift weapons of opportunity, the victim's immediate environment or firearms.
3. The most effective self-defense techniques require minimal strength and take advantage of leverage and knowledge of vital targets on the body.
4. Effective self-defense techniques are simple and easy to learn and can include kicking, stomping, choking, grappling, gouging, poking, biting and any other method that gets the job done.

A basic self-defense program should include awareness training where students are taught specific methods for avoiding and recognizing potentially dangerous situations or individuals before trouble starts. As in medicine, prevention is the best medicine. If a student can avoid a possible assault or confrontation, that is the best self defense of all. You want to learn the psychology of defending yourself even before trouble actually starts.

For those situations where alertness or psychology are not sufficient to deal with the problem, basic self-defense training should include escape maneuvers for the most common types of grabs, chokes and holds, more advanced defensive moves to combat punches and kicks, and counters for armed attacks.

In a purely self-defense program you will not be taught to become a martial artist in the traditional sense with belts and ranks. You are simply learning a vocabulary of self defense techniques with which you can respond to situations that you are likely to encounter.

In addition to escape techniques, you should learn techniques and drills for striking and disabling an assailant. In the domain of self defense, techniques typically fall into one of two categories: destructive, disabling techniques and non-destructive controlling techniques. Destructive techniques are intended to maim or kill. They are only used as a desperate last resort after first attempting to diffuse the situation with non-destructive, controlling techniques which allow the victim to escape, but ultimately leave the assailant free of permanent injuries. Below are some important principles of self-defense and combat situations that you must keep in mind as you train.

## Universal Principles of Combat

1. Combat is fluid dynamic and messy
2. Combat and assaults are totally unscripted, unpredictable and unstructured.
3. Effective self-defense cannot not follow pre-scripted sequences of movements. It must be fluid and adaptable; incorporating various tactics, methods and strategies and the will to survive.
4. No two instances of personal combat are exactly alike. Each situation is unique with all its factors and variables.
5. Core movements in a self-defense situation must utilize gross motor movements.
6. Focused, controlled anger can help you survive; paralyzing fear, distraction and hesitation will get you killed.

Continue and learn more advanced self-defense techniques and then consider training in a traditional martial art. Continuation in a traditional martial arts belt system will significantly enhance your physical conditioning, skill levels, confidence and knowledge, however, there are a number of self-defense options in most metropolitan areas.

## Reality Check: Today's Combat

1. Crime occurs in the nicest of neighborhoods and to the nicest people. The sooner you get that the better off you will be.
2. You need to learn to protect yourself from violent, vicious criminals. Pure muscular strength is not self-defense.
3. You are the only person whom you can count on to take responsibility to ensure your safety and survival.
4. There simply aren't enough police around to protect you. Self-protection is your job and you need to know what to do in different scenarios such as a shooting spree or one-on-one assault.
5. There is no complete guarantee of safety, but self-defense training can give you an edge and improve your chances of survival in a violent assault.

Red Man classes are popular. Essentially, these classes involve a human target, the aggressor, dressed in martial arts protective padded gear from head to toe. Class members learn basic strikes, punches, kicks and the like and are able to practice against a live aggressor who attempts to attack them. The quality of these classes varies greatly, but check and see what is available in your area. If you are serious about learning some very basic concepts and techniques quickly to kick start your skills, this may be an option prior to more structure learning in something like a traditional martial arts school.

Krav Maga – the Israeli system of self-defense is not a traditional martial art. While some Krav Maga schools do incorporate a belt system, this is not how the system was originally structured. Nonetheless, there are a number of variants of Krav Maga including Commando Krav Maga and so forth. There are a growing number of Krav Maga organizations that have splintered off from the original system and some of them offer instructor certification programs. Check your local area for options or even consult your local police or sheriff department to see what they recommend.

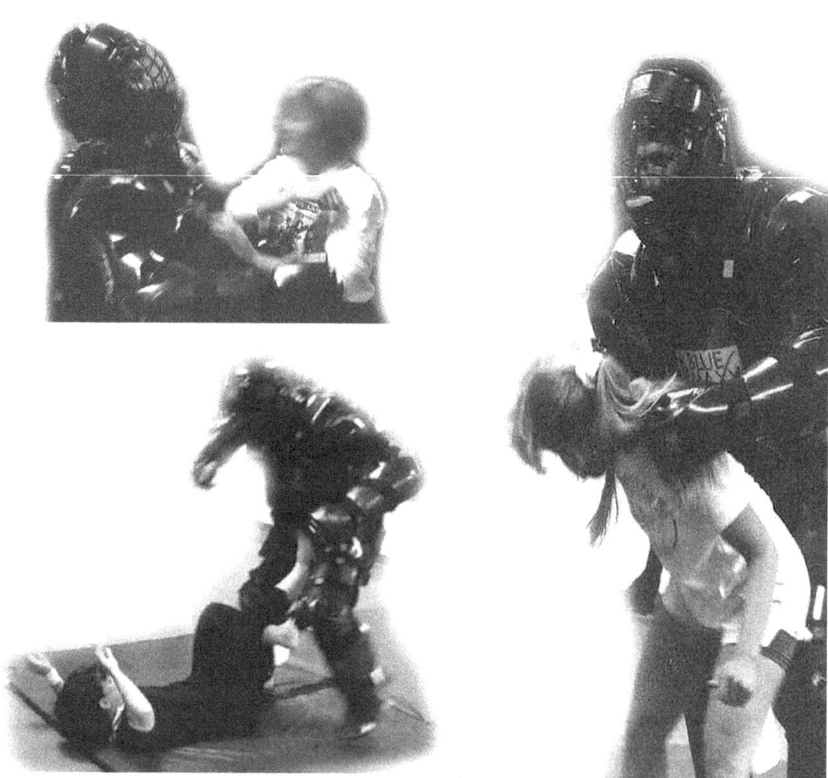

*A self-defense class where participants strike a heavily padded assailant in realistic assault situations*

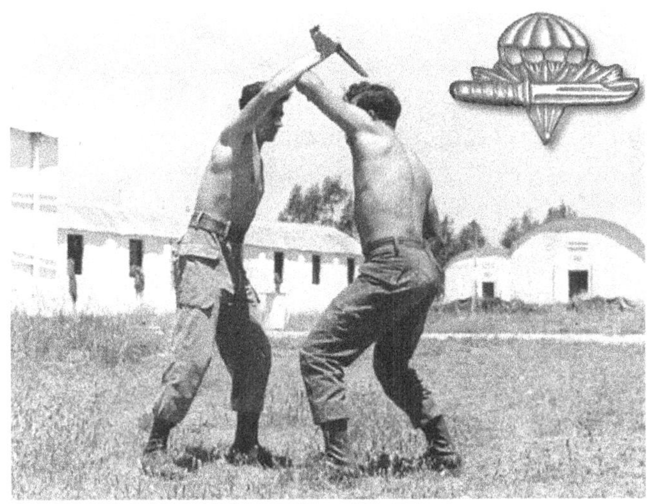

*Israeli Commandos practice Krav Maga*

## Realism

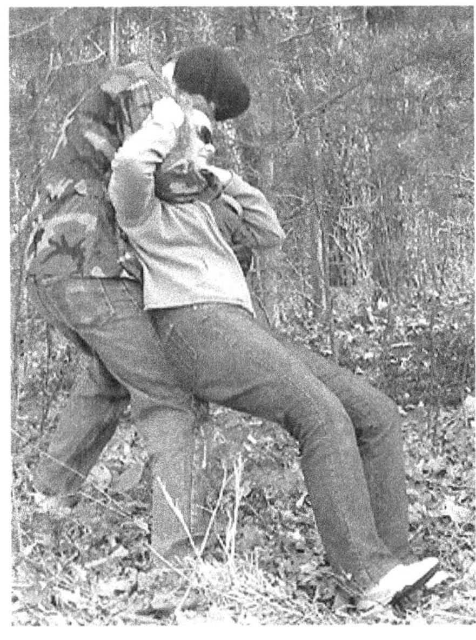

The more realistic the training experience ... the less shocking reality will seem. Part of varying your training is practicing for realism. Take your training seriously. If it is a joke or becomes too much of a social gathering, you will be easily surprised or overwhelmed in a real situation. Some schools of martial arts practice in swamps, rain, and all types of terrain and environments. Martial arts are a war fighting skill where realism is a key ingredient in training. Part of the reason for the diversity and variation in training is to introduce different realistic elements. A curious thing happens when you make a training drill very realistic, you become uncomfortable. In the Marine Corps Martial Arts Program (MCMAP) and in many traditional martial arts schools across the world, some aspects of the training are conducted in realistic settings, rain, snow, and sand, in shallow streams or ponds and in uneven terrain. Some training is at night and all of these conditions are intended to simulate reality and the conditions in which a student, soldier or law enforcement officer might find themselves having to apply their martial arts skills.

At United Karate we used to take students out into the parking light occasionally and have them dressed in street clothes. We would have other senior in students hiding behind cars and positioned in other hiding spots ready to leap out and simulate an assault on the students in training so that they could get used to working in confined spaces such as between cars or at night with limited lighting and visibility. The point was to make the training a challenge and then see how the students performed. Every one appreciated the dose of reality. Reality isn't always pleasant, but reality is what you are training for. Being uncomfortable is a good thing. Get used to it in training so that you will not be surprised if it happens for real.

## *Grappling and Chokes*

Some styles of martial arts include grappling techniques others exclude grappling. If you are in tight quarters and are unable to execute a kick or a strong punch, you may have to use grappling techniques. Grappling, with its holds, arm-bars, joint manipulation and joint locks should be part of your martial arts training. It makes you a more robust opponent and understanding at least some basic grappling will help you defend against it as well.

Most fights begin as shoving matches or as grappling or wrestling situations and yet many traditional styles ignore this, why? Grappling can be a little more involved than basic kicking and punching. Some styles argue that as long as you can keep your opponent at a distance, you can kick or punch, but what if you are caught by surprise with a grab from behind. This is a grappling situation. Without knowledge of grappling, you are at a loss and may panic when your limited training fails you because you have not prepared for such a situation.

Learn grappling, it is essential for close range fighting. Grappling also has legal advantages. If you can subdue an opponent without causing damage, you may not be liable for injuries that you might cause by other, more destructive techniques such as kicks or strikes.

## *Kicking*

There are many beautiful and deadly kicks in different styles of martial arts. Like grappling, punching and joint manipulation, kicking has its place and it should have a place in your library of techniques. Kicks need not be head-level to be effective. The most effective kicks are those, which you can deliver without putting your balance or footing at risk. The more unstable the surface, on which you are standing, such as ice, snow, gravel, the lower the kicks should be. Aim for vital targets, groin, side of the knee, thighs, ankles, bridge of the foot.

You can cause much damage with kicks below the belt. You need not risk falling or being pushed off balance by trying to kick someone in the head. Conversely, with enough experience and expertise, you can deliver high kicks to the head or upper body with devastating power if you are certain of the conditions, but higher kicks still entail higher risk. Timing, distance, power, speed, experience and environment are all key factors, not to mention the nature of your opponent.

As with all other techniques, learn a wide variety of kicks, preferably the more practical ones. Learn which targets are most appropriate for which kicks and what situations are most appropriate. Practice kicking drills for timing, speed, flexibility, power and distance. Keep these skills sharp, as with all other techniques, they are part of your total arsenal. Have them ready and waiting. You will know the right time to use them.

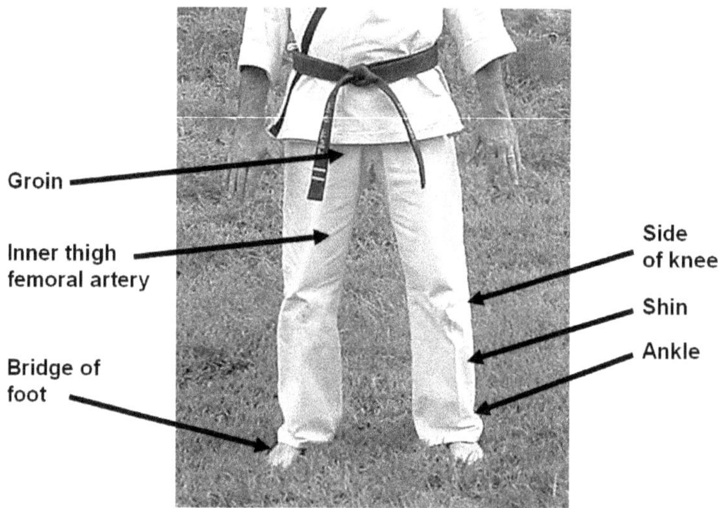


*Common targets below the belt*

Low kicks are the most effective. Kicks that are waist-level or below are safer for the person executing the kick. A higher kicking target will result in the kicker being unable to generate as much force as with a lower kick due to the effects of gravity. The kicker will also have less balance. Therefore the most powerful and stable kicks are those that aim for waist level and below.

## Hand Techniques

There is a wide variety of hand techniques available to the martial artist. You are not limited to simply using the fist to punch. You can use hand techniques for effective strikes to the eyes, throat, nose, groin and other vital points. Every martial arts style has its favored set of techniques. Learning a good variety of them will improve your overall arsenal and give you additional options in

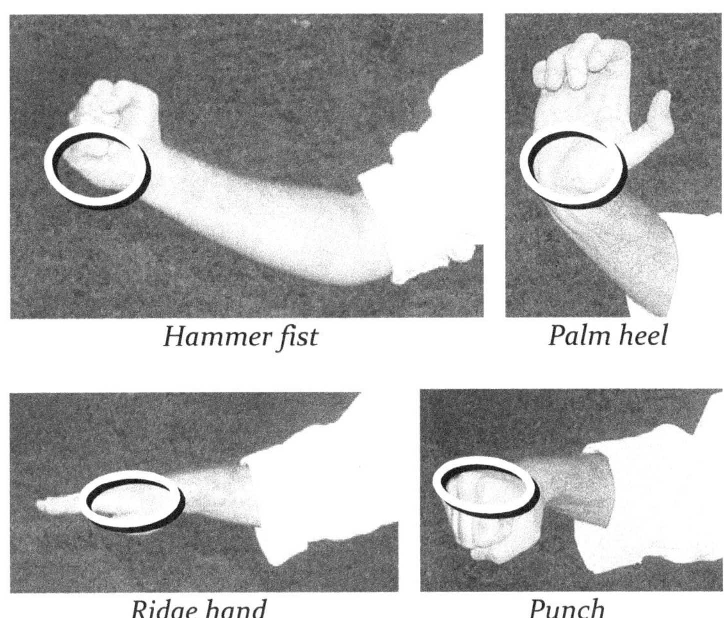

*Hammer fist* *Palm heel*

*Ridge hand* *Punch*

*Various weapons of the hand. Circles indicate the strike point of the weapon.*

There are also many uses for the elbow. Elbow strikes can be used to strike the stomach, the face, jaw and the spine and other targets.

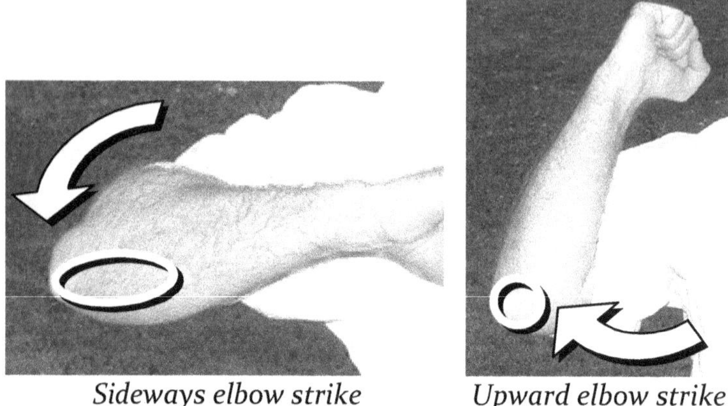

*Sideways elbow strike* *Upward elbow strike*

*Elbow strikes: Strike points are circled. Arrows indicate the path of movement of the arm.*

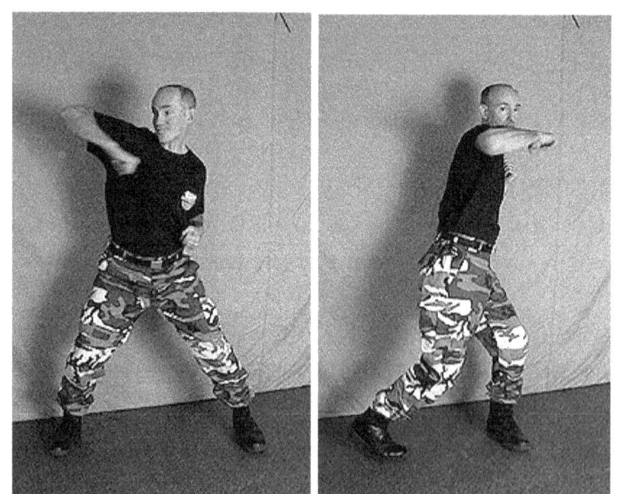

*Left: A front elbow strike*
*Right: A horizontal sweeping elbow strike*

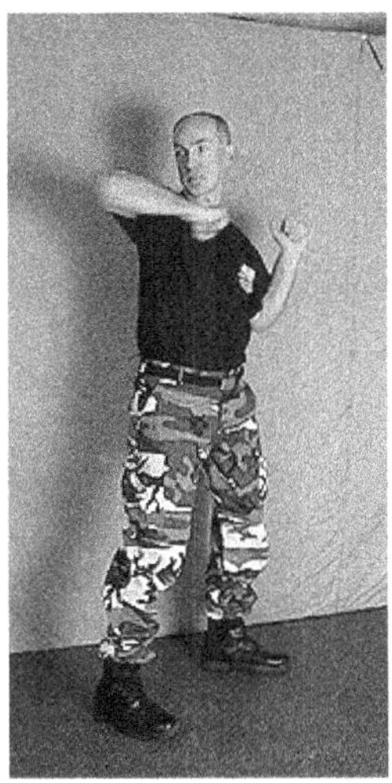

*A back elbow strike*

## *Ground Fighting*

Most fights end up on the ground. When they do, what happens next depends upon who is the better ground fighter. If you have no training in ground fighting and your opponent has even one single effective technique in his arsenal that he is able to execute against you, you are at a serious disadvantage.

As I mentioned with grappling, you must learn these things. Ground fighting is a part of grappling. Grappling can take place either standing or it can take place on the ground. Many of the same grappling techniques that work in an upright manner will also work on the ground. This is your starting point. You will also notice that you can apply many of the grappling techniques from the kata while you are pinned on the ground. You are simply in a different position and the techniques might require some slight modification, but this gives you a good starting point.

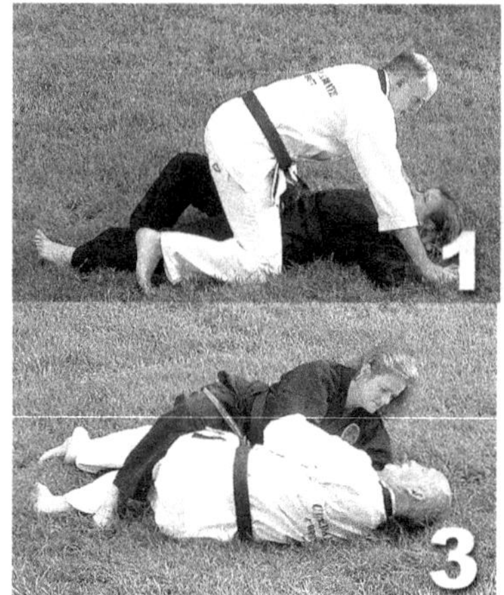


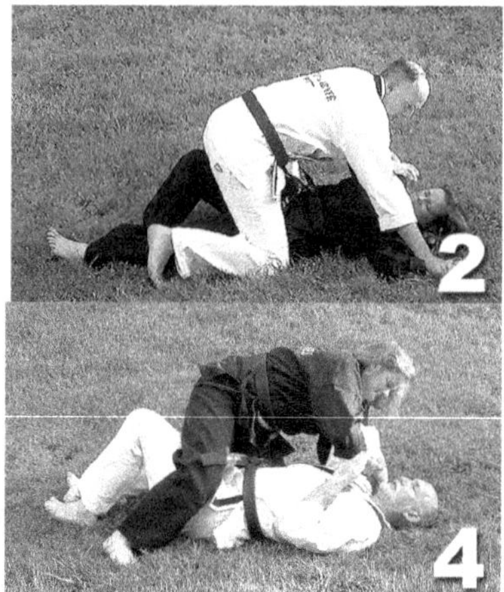


*The defender, in black, is pinned down, but uses a dissolve to the bone, followed by a chop to the elbow with a hand wedge to stress the elbow joint providing leverage to roll her opponent over while maintaining a folded arm bar for control.*

Your goal in all training is to reduce or eliminate disadvantages. Give yourself advantages by making your training as comprehensive as possible. Study fighting techniques and methods for all types of opponents and situations even if they are not officially part of your specific style or curriculum. They exist and someone else may use them against you. Prepare yourself. Even if you have not studied a particular type of opponent or situation in detail, the mere fact that you have diverse training experience will likely help you adapt to a new situation more rapidly than someone who is strictly traditional and staid in his or her training and thinking.

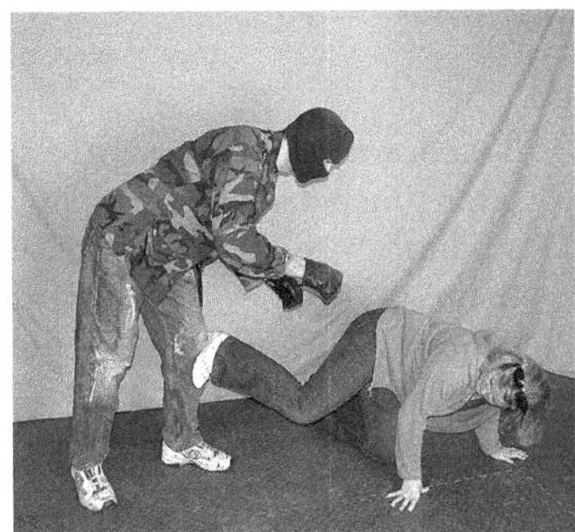
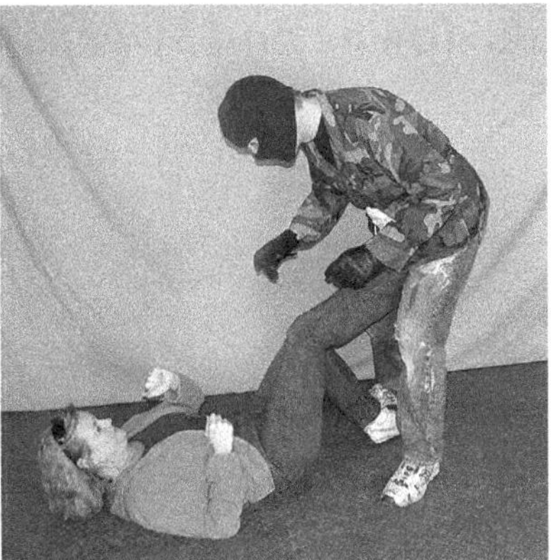

*To survive you must be able to fight from any position*

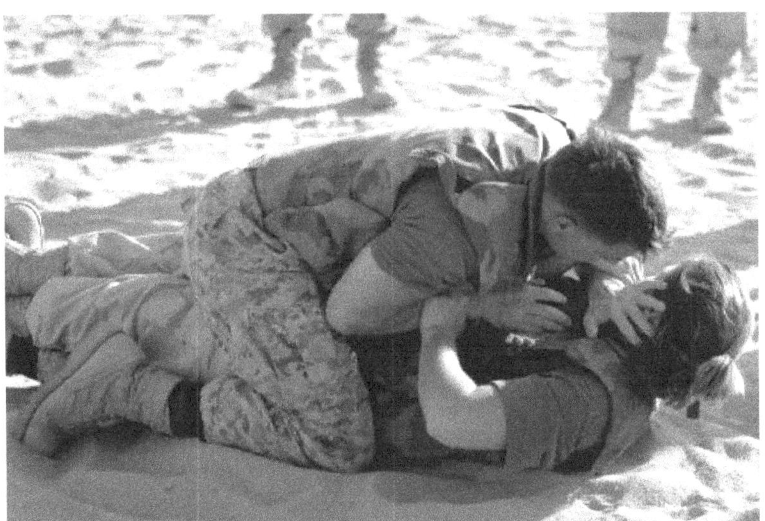

*U.S. Marines practice ground fighting in the sand as part of the Marine Corps Martial Arts Program.*

## Takedowns and Sweeps

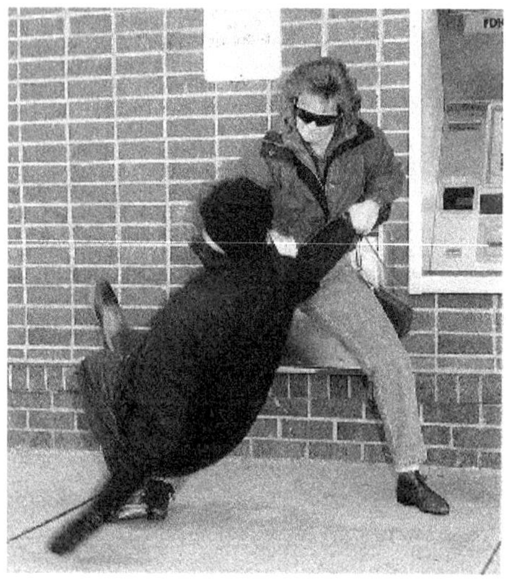

Takedowns and sweeps are often included in grappling studies. You can accomplish them from grappling maneuvers. They are useful because they can put your opponent down and reduce the potential threat.

If your opponent is not skilled in ground fighting and your sweep or takedown brings both of you down in a flurry of grabs, you will still have the advantage, because by bringing them down to the ground where you are experienced, you have just brought them down into your territory. This gives you the advantage, but only if you are properly trained.

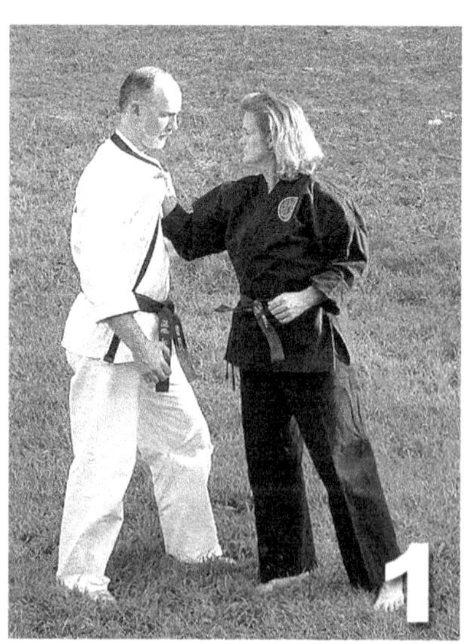



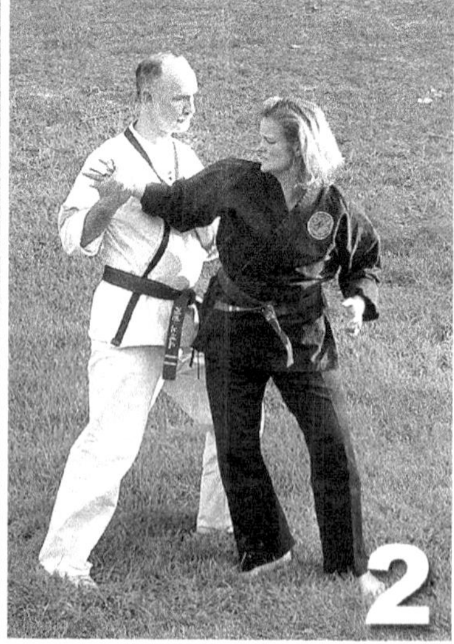

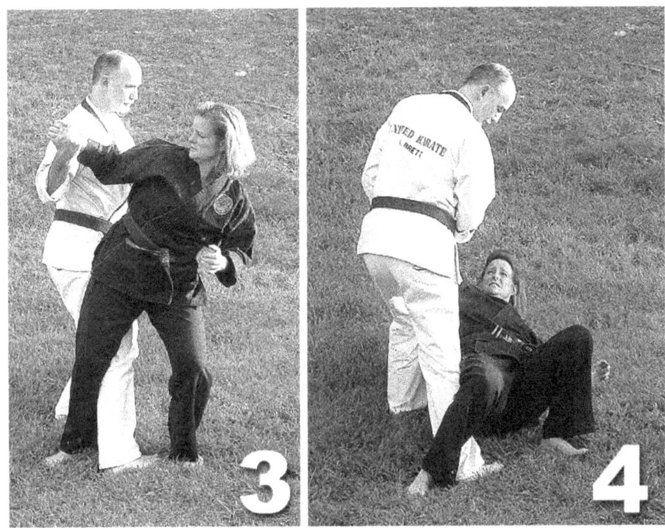


*The defender, in white, uses a wrist manipulation to twist the opponent over and down to the ground.*

## Classical Weapons

Many schools and instructors have no experience with or knowledge of weapons. They assume that all martial arts involve hand-to-hand combat. This could not be further from the truth. Weapons techniques represent at least half of martial arts.

There are dozens of primary martial arts weapons and hundreds of less common, but nonetheless useful and effective weapons. Weapons and their techniques have evolved over the centuries side by side with unarmed techniques.

If for no other reason than to preserve their heritage, you should study weapons. However, there are many other reasons for the study of classical weapons. All well designed martial arts weapons are an extension of the users hand or arm. They are designed or used in such a manner as to become a part of the person carrying them.

The very soul of the Japanese Samurai, for example, is the Katana - the long sword. The Samurai went nowhere without this blade. The Japanese Ninja, on the other hand, were well versed in a wide array of weapons and means of waging warfare with them; everything from hand-made explosives to grappling hooks to short, straight versions of the Samurai Katana.

The study of weapons can begin with intermediate students. At the intermediate level, students have begun to develop the rudiments of knowledge about movement, open hand technique and physical conditioning. At this point, it is possible to begin your study of weapons so that you may begin to see how to integrate a weapon into their arsenal of techniques and how the weapon becomes a natural extension of you. It will also be important to you as an intermediate student to begin to understand how to block and deflect various types of strikes or blows with primitive weapons such as a club or even a pool queue.

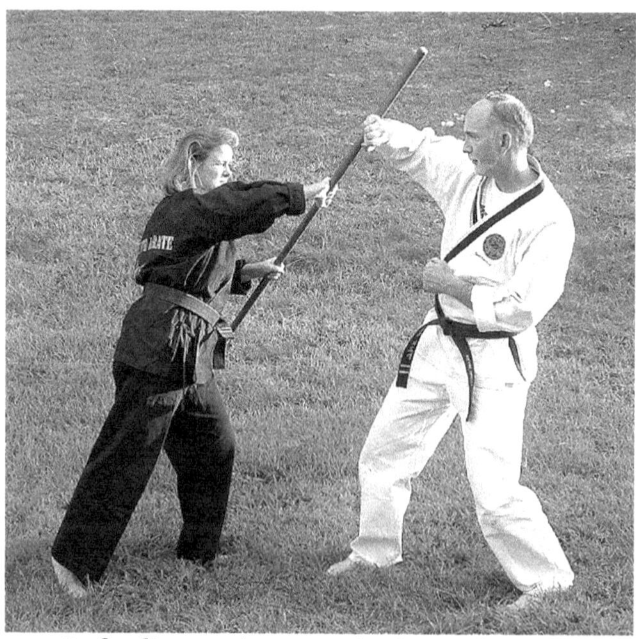

*Defending against a strike from a bo-staff.*

You can begin to see how to move with and without a weapon. You can begin to understand movement and body mechanics better through the study of the motion of a weapon. You also begin to understand how to use the striking or blocking power of the weapon to cause damage in the same way that you begin to learn how to use the striking or blocking ability of their arms or legs.

| Common Classical Martial Arts Weapons | |
|---|---|
| | **Name:** Nunchukas<br>**Purpose:** Originally used for beating stalks of rice. For combat they can be swung in many directions with enough force to crush a skull. |
| | **Name:** Ninto (Japanese Ninja Sword)<br>**Purpose:** Used by Ninja as an inexpensive, medium version of the Samurai sword. |
| | **Name:** Kamas (and their blade covers)<br>**Purpose:** Used like a scythe to harvest rice, but also used in martial arts to slice, stab and chop. |
| | **Name:** Pair of Tonfas<br>**Purpose:** Used to grind rice originally, but in martial arts either end can be used to strike and holding the handle, the length can be used to shield the arm. |

| | |
|---|---|
| 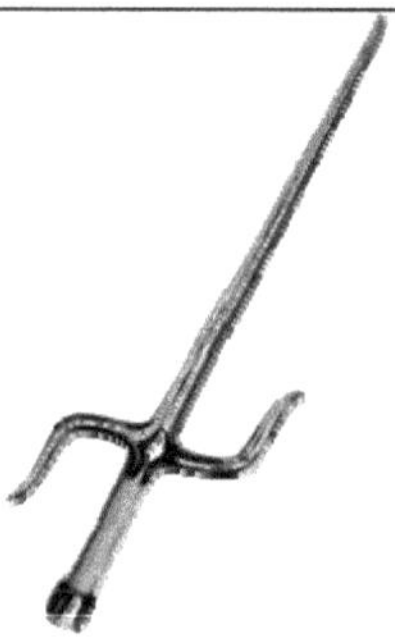 | **Name:** Sai<br>**Purpose:** Used originally as a pin for an ox-cart, in martial arts it is used to trap the blade of a sword during a downward strike or to jab or stab the opponent. The handle of the sai can be used to strike and the length can be used like the tonfa to shield the forearm. |
| 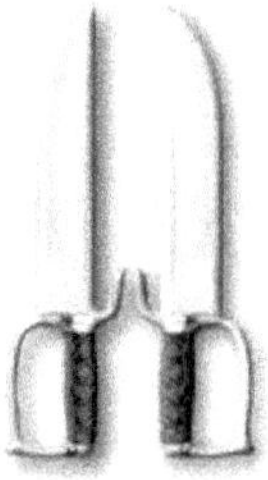 | **Name:** Chinese Butterfly Swords<br>**Purpose:** Often used to cut meat, they are effective in slicing or stabbing the opponent. |
| 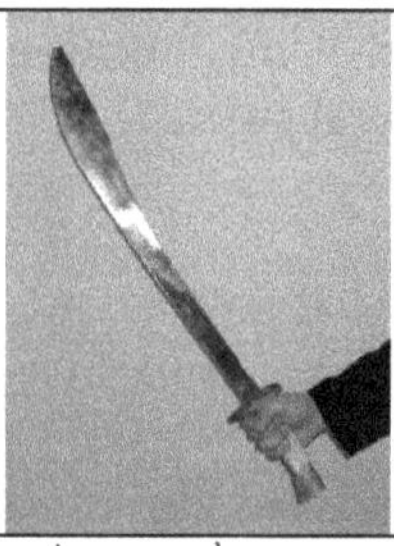 | **Name:** Chinese Saber<br>**Purpose:** Used for general combat |
| 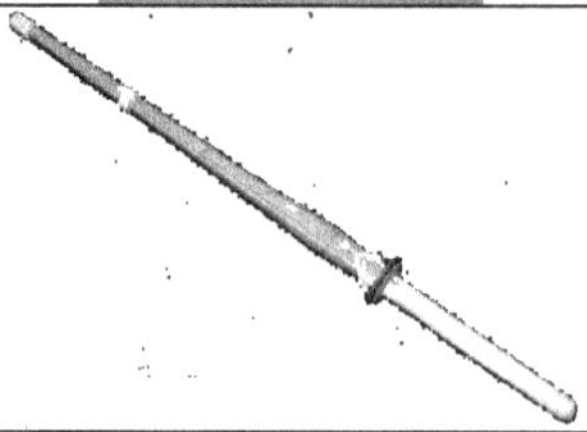 | **Name:** Shinai<br>**Purpose:** A practice sword made of split bamboo. It is used in Japanese Kendo. |
| 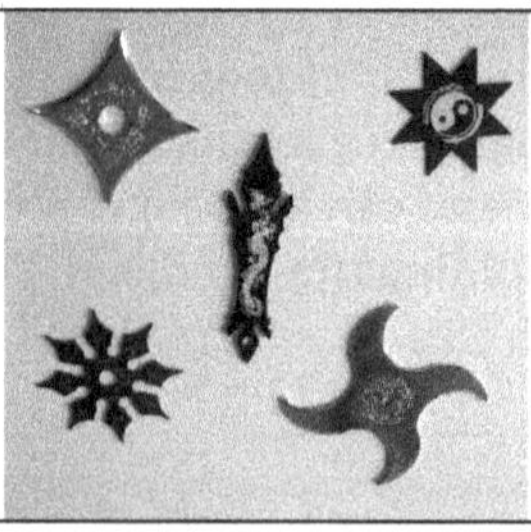 | **Name:** Shurikens<br>**Purpose:** These are throwing stars used to penetrate the target. They can pierce a human skull or eviscerate soft tissue. |

Many common martial arts weapons were derived from everyday objects in the countries and times in which they evolved. Farmers used nunchakus to beat stalks of rice. Rice farmers used kamas to cut rice. Farmers often used Sais as pins for ox carts. The bo-staff had many everyday uses such as carrying pails of water or dirt.

Typical martial arts weapons may not be legal to carry today as they were in previous centuries, but through their study, the martial artist can learn to adapt and utilize everyday objects of this century for the same purposes - self-defense. This is where it is important to study weapons of opportunity.

## *Weapons of Opportunity*

Weapons of opportunity refer to the employment of everyday objects as weapons in your own self-defense. Examples include:

**Weapons of Opportunity**

- Canes
- Umbrellas
- Flashlights
- Clubs
- Spray cans and liquids
- Dirt/Dust/Gravel/Rocks
- Pens/Pencils
- Fire extinguishers
- Belts
- Dinner knives
- Dinner plates
- Pots and pans
- Coffee mugs, and many more

Weapons of opportunity can be used for self-defense and those things around you like a kitchen knife, a cane or an umbrella can be used against an assailant to gain an advantage.

Items in your house, workplace or school can be used as weapons. Look around the house and take inventory of various rooms, discuss with your spouse or children how items such as a skillet can be used to strike an attacker in the head or face. Other items such as kitchen steak knives or cooking knives can be used. A vase in the dining room or living room can be used to hit the assailant on the head. Dinner plates, beer bottles, wine bottles and countless other items can be used as means of self-defense. Always think of how the weapon could be used to strike vital targets on the attacker such as face, eyes, throat, nose, ears, groin, knees or ankles.

## *Effective Defense*

Martial arts systems are built upon many techniques for protecting against and causing temporary or permanent pain, damage or injury to an aggressor. For these techniques to be effective in self-defense situation, the martial artist must know what damage a technique can inflict on an opponent. Most martial arts schools do not teach this because their instructors do not know it themselves. Knowledge of the medical implications of various martial arts techniques is crucial for effective self-defense.

Knowledge of basic anatomy and the physiology of movement is important in helping the martial artist learn how to execute the technique so that it will have the desired medical consequence. This is not a pleasant subject, but neither is assault, murder or rape, which of course is what a martial artist hopes to prevent or avoid.

## *Child Safety*

Self-defense for children is a challenging subject. There are books and videos available that teach techniques, but the reality is that an adult male or female of even average strength can physically overcome a young child. At United Karate we began teaching self-defense techniques to students beginning at age twelve because this is typically the midst of the middle-school years where children are often the meanest to each other. In elementary school, what few physical altercations might occur can be dealt with by using the basic kicks, punches or blocks taught by most martial arts styles. Of course this is only a last resort when the child feels physically threatened by another child of approximately the same age.

To address the issue of responding to a much larger, stronger child or adult assailant, I prefer to focus on one very simple acronym as a memory and training aid. **Fire and G.E.T. Out.** (Groin, Eyes, Throat). It's an incredibly simple approach. First, other adults generally will not turn their head to notice if another child is screaming for help or yelling "stop!" We're simply exposed to too many instances of children playing around or joking or simply becoming angry with each other to respond every time we hear this plea for help. When someone yells "Fire" however, we don't hear that everyday and our subconscious is programmed from a very early age to fear fire and its effects. That typically makes a much more effective plea for help.

The G.E.T portion tells your child what they must do; strike the assailants, groin, eyes and throat in any order with any weapon, punch, chop or poke they can. Strike one or all of these targets many times, strike hard and strike fast. Even the strongest adult can be distracted, injured or disabled if your child focuses on those three targets. Your child's hands or arms may be pinned or held, but at some point during the assault they can hopeful have a second where they may be free to strike – that is the chance they must watch for. It might just save their life!

It is also important for children to be taught concepts of street awareness and playground safety as well as school safety and what to do in tragic situations such as school shootings. I do not have space here to go into a treatment of these topics, but the resources block in this chapter contains several excellent books on these topics.

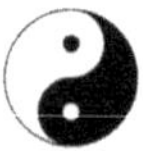

## Resources

**Books**:

1. Surviving A School Shooting – Loren Christensen
2. Warrior Wisdom: The Warrior's Path – Dr. Bohdi Sanders
3. Surviving Armed Assaults: A Martial Artists Guide to Weapons, Street Violence, and Countervailing Force – Lawrence Kane
4. The Little Black Book of Violence: What Every Young Man Needs to Know About Fighting – Lawrence Kane, Kris Wilder
5. How to Win a Fight: A Guide to Surviving Violence – Lawrence Kane, Kris Wilder
6. Achieving Kicking Excellence Series (Combat Applications) Vols 11 – 20 – Shawn Kovacich
7. Solo Training 2: The Martial Artist's Guide to Building the Core for Stronger, Faster and More Effective Grappling, Kicking and Punching (No. 2) - Lawren Christensen
8. Girl Power: Self-Defense for Teens – B. Konzak

# Chapter 4

# Key Martial Arts Training Concepts

*"Lifting weights and running marathons is fun, but that will not keep you safe. Training for real situations helps you practice the appropriate response."*

## What's it Like in Martial Arts Class?

Well, every school is different. There are many similarities. Some schools are quite disciplined and formalized, following traditional martial arts training methods and other schools may be more casual and not even concerned with tradition.

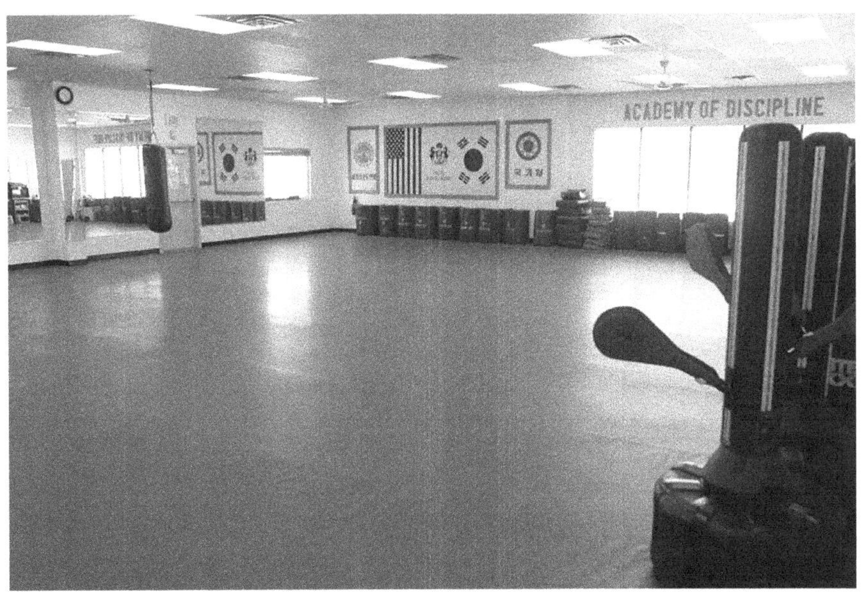

Here is an example of how a fairly traditional martial arts class might go: Before students enter the classroom or workout room (Dojang in Korean, or Dojo in Japanese and Okinawan), they should remove their shoes (socks are often ok, but may be bothersome when trying to move around). This is oriental custom and tradition. It also helps to keep the carpet or wood floor from getting dirty quickly. Shoes can be put on again once the student has returned to the waiting area or lobby. (Frankly, working in your bare feet helps condition your feet!)

As you enter or leave the Dojang, it is customary to bow to the flags on the wall. Usually you will see a United States flag and a Korean flag (the homeland of Tae Kwon Do) or a Japanese flag (the homeland of many Japanese styles of martial arts). The United States flag symbolizes our great nation; while the other flags represent the home countries of whatever martial arts are taught. Bowing has no religious connotation. It is simply a way of showing respect for the law of the land and the great institutions of the United States and the art of Tae Kwon Do or whatever is taught in the school.

Typically at the beginning of class students will line up and bow first to the flags, then to the instructor(s). This tradition teaches humility and respect to the student. It is an acknowledgement of the superior knowledge and skill in martial arts represented by the presence of the instructors. This honor and respect will be your right to earn and maintain as you climb to the black belt level and beyond.

After bowing, class begins by reciting some form of student creed. The Student Creed describes the ethics of martial arts and serves as a constant reminder to students and instructors alike that martial arts are to be used for defensive purposes only.

All black belts should be addressed as Sir or Ma'am. This reinforces respect and humility, key ingredients to success in the martial arts and elsewhere. Before addressing a Black Belt a student should go to attention and bow before asking a question or making a statement. How formal and serious your school is about this martial etiquette varies greatly from school to school and instructor to instructor.

All kicks, punches and chops should ideally be executed with a fierce yell. The yell is normally referred to as a "kiai". Yelling at the time of impact helps to focus the power of the mind and body upon the task of striking the opponent. The more concentrated the strike, the more effective it will be. The yell also serves to distract, scare or startle your opponent and disturb their concentration.

Tae Kwon Do and other **MARTIAL ARTS TECHNIQUES ARE STRICKTLY FOR DEFENSE ONLY**. Martial arts are not be used outside the classroom unless the student is entering a martial arts tournament or demonstration or in a true self-defense situation where there is no escape or other peaceful resolution or alternative.

**Martial arts are never to be used to threaten, provoke or physically harm another person. Martial arts techniques should be used as a last resort only, in physically threatening situations.**

Some classes begin with a series of warm up exercises to get the blood pumping and warm up the muscles. The increased blood flow also helps stimulate mental awareness and prepare the student for learning. Physical conditioning is an important part of martial arts. Everyone is not expected to become an Olympic caliber athlete, but improving strength, cardiovascular endurance and flexibility all aid the student in preparing for competition or for real-life self-defense situations. The better prepared and better conditioned individual will typically fare better against one of lesser abilities and that is the goal. Some schools, however, will expect the student to enter the class already warmed up and prepared to learn.

After warm ups, classes will sometimes enter meditation position. Again, there is no religious connotation to the meditation that we practice. Meditation simply gives the student a few moments to return the heart rate to a normal level before stretching. In meditation, the student should clear their mind of all thoughts but their training and how to improve themselves.

You should concentrate on positive goals, be it improving a particular kicking technique or picturing yourself progressing to the next level belt. Practice visualizing yourself being successful in your martial arts endeavors, whether the goal is to loose weight and get in better physical conditions, or to improve sparring techniques, so that you can increase your chances of winning a tournament. Meditation is a period of focusing and self-motivation. Many sports trainers and athletes agree that visualization of goals is essential to achieving them.

Cross training is encouraged. You should participate in other sports and developmental physical activities. Jogging, walking, swimming, biking, weight-lifting, and many other sports help to contribute to the level of conditioning, health and overall self-satisfaction of the student.

Many students will find that after a year or more of martial arts training that other sports or physical activities that they had engage in previously are improved because of their increased levels of conditioning, coordination, flexibility and strength from martial arts.

As with anything in life, ***moderation is the key to success.*** You should try to maintain a consistent training and exercise schedule. It is better to train three times per week in martial arts or jogging and do so consistently, than to train seven days per week for one month and then not a all for a period of time. No matter how much you may enjoy something, moderation and consistency will help prevent burnout and ultimately produce far superior results.

## Rules of the School

1. Students and instructors should bow when entering or leaving the Dojang.
2. Students must be properly attired in their official uniform for all classes. The uniform should be kept clean and neatly pressed. Rips, holes or tears should be mended or the uniform replaced.
3. The uniform should not be worn without a belt unless the student is at the no-belt level. Belts should be treated with respect and as a symbol of rank and achievement. Belts should NEVER be washed as a reminder of the hard work and sweat that was required to earn them.
4. When adjusting the uniform or belt, the student or instructor should turn away from the flags in the front of the classroom as a sign of respect.
5. Students should be considerate of those around them and observe good personal hygiene. That includes bathing and wearing deodorants to keep from offending others. Perfume or colognes should NOT be worn, or should be worn sparingly for the same reason.

   All Nails should be trimmed for safety since martial arts is a contact activity. This reduces the chances of the student scratching or cutting another person or themselves.
6. Students must not wear jewelry, watches or sharp objects when working out. These items can catch, cut or scratch others.
7. When students are in the Dojang they should be focused on improving their martial arts skills and knowledge. That means that they should be practicing, stretching or helping other students. Students should not engage in loud, distracting, talking or laughing. This is in consideration of the instructors, the other students and the spirit of the martial arts.
8. Students should not eat, drink or chew gum in the workout areas.
9. Students should be courteous and helpful to each other and especially to the instructors. Students should offer to help

instructors set up equipment, pads, mats, etc. if they see that the instructor could use some help.

10. Students should never use their martial arts skill except in the aid of a friend, loved one or for self-defense. To do otherwise violates the ethics of the martial arts and is considered a felony in most jurisdictions.

## *Uniform and Equipment Care*

If your style of martial arts uses fairly traditional uniforms such as those in Korean and Japanese styles there are a few useful tips to caring for these uniforms that will make them last longer and stay looking good.

Most martial arts uniforms are made entirely of cotton. Even though some manufacturers claim that their uniform is preshrunk, use caution, especially with commercial dryers. The following tips will help with care and maintenance of uniforms and sparring gear.

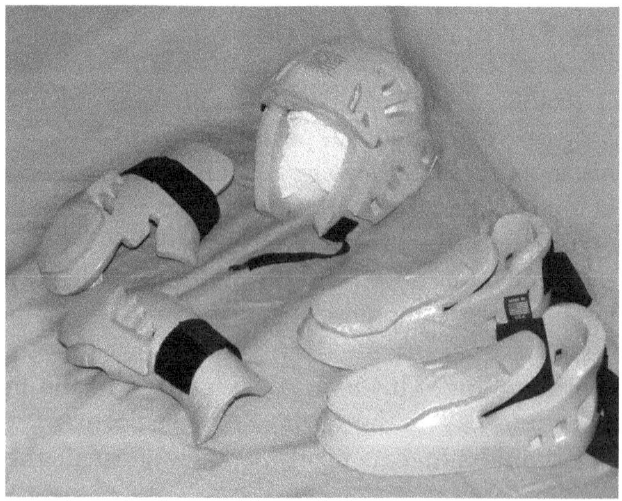

*A typical set of dipped-foam sparring gear*

## Uniform Care and Maintenance Tips

1. Use a spray cleaner or other cleaning supplement to spot clean the uniform before putting it into the washer.

2. Wash it with hot water, but use a non-bleach detergent. A detergent that bleaches the uniform will also bleach the school patch or any other patches.

3. Pull the arms and legs inside out before putting it into the washing. This will prevent the patches or silkscreen or embroidered logos and lettering from becoming snagged or torn.

4. Uniform drying instructions
   Follow the manufactures instructions on the uniform. In general, it is best to air dry or dry on low heat. Drying is when the uniform is most likely to shrink. After two washings most uniforms will have finished shrinking and will remain that size unless dried in high heat.

5. Uniform fitting instructions
   After the uniform has been washed two or three times the pants can then be hemmed to the proper length. It is a good idea, especially for children, to hem the paths up and keep any extra material rather than cutting off the excess. This will leave you with material to work with if the pants ever shrink or need lengthening.

   Generally the top can have the sleeves rolled up neatly to about the elbow or top part of the forearm. The sleeves should not be above elbow since the uniform also offers protection from rug burns or scratches from sparring.

   Traditional pants should be lengthened or shortened so that they come down and cover the ankle. Again, this acts as protection. Pants that are drooping over the bridge of the foot can be dangerous and cause the student to trip and fall.

## Sparring Equipment Care Tips

The useful lifetime of the equipment you use to spar will vary with each student and the specific manufacturer and construction of the equipment and it depends up how often you spar and how well you care for your gear. Most commercial schools use foam padded equipment that is dipped in plastic one or more times. This offers ample protection from kicks and punches and helps absorb much of the direct impact. Injury can still occur, but will be mitigated by wearing of appropriate gear. Some schools adhere to completely traditional practices and use no gear at all. This is one reason you will need to visit several schools of different styles to decide which is your cup of green tea!

1. Don't leave sparring equipment in the cold or heat. Many times students leave their equipment in the car in the winder or summer. In the cold weather, sparring equipment will become hard or even brittle and loose much of its flexibility and shock absorbing qualities. This reduces the level of protection available when sparring.
2. In the summer, equipment left in a hot area such as a car will partially melt or shrivel. The same problem occurs where the equipment looses some of its shock absorbing ability. Sometimes equipment left in the heat will tear more easily because the thin layer of latex covering the padding has grown even thinner in the heat.
3. Whenever sparring equipment becomes moderately torn, hard, inflexible, chipped or otherwise damaged, it should be replaced as soon as possible. Otherwise it is not offering the full level of protection it was designed to provide.
4. Wipe down the equipment after sparring. If you are interested in extending the life of your equipment you should use a towel and wipe down the gear after sparring. The salt in sweat will cause the equipment to begin to deteriorate over time unless it is wiped down.
5. Periodically rinse the equipment. Put all of the gear into a bathtub with luke warm water and mild, liquid dish soap. Gently wash and rinse the equipment in luke warm water. Once per month is a reasonable interval depending upon how much the equipment gets used. Remember, hot or cold water will have the same effect

as leaving it in the heat or cold.

6. Mouth Guards
   Mouth guards must be suitable for martial arts training. This means that mouth guards designed for other sports such as football are not adequate. A minimum of a single mouth guard is recommended. Double mouth guards cover upper and lower teeth offer additional protection. If you choose to wear a football style mouth guard with the long rubber tether used to connect the mouth guard to the football helmet, then you must cut off the tether so that only the mouth guard is left. Often parents think a child is less likely to loose their mouth guard if it is attached to their head guard. The idea is good except that when sparring, a finger or hand could catch the tether and rip the mouthpiece from the student's mouth risking possible injury.

   If a student is using a martial arts headgear with the football style bars attached (usually for students who wear glasses) then a football style mouth guard is permitted since the bars are in front of the mouth for protection. Before using a mouth guard it must be molded to fit the wearer. Follow the manufacturer's instructions and make sure you have a good fit. If it doesn't quite fit correctly, most guards can be remolded by repeating the process.

7. Wearing Equipment
   All equipment should be securely attached before beginning to spar. Rib guards can be worn either on top of the uniform or underneath. Shin guards, optional knee pads and groin cups should be worn underneath the uniform to offer maximum range of movement and protection. Groin cups should never be worn on top of the uniform pants.

## *Setting Physical Fitness Goals*

Other important goals which martial arts can help us accomplish are fitness goals. While we are learning to defend ourselves or enjoying the sport and competition of karate, our bodies are also reaping the benefits of the physical activity of the martial arts.

**HEALTH WARNING: As with all physical activity, before beginning a program of any physical activity, visit a physician to discuss your planned activities and have your overall health assessed to ensure that you are healthy enough to engage in your new activities.**

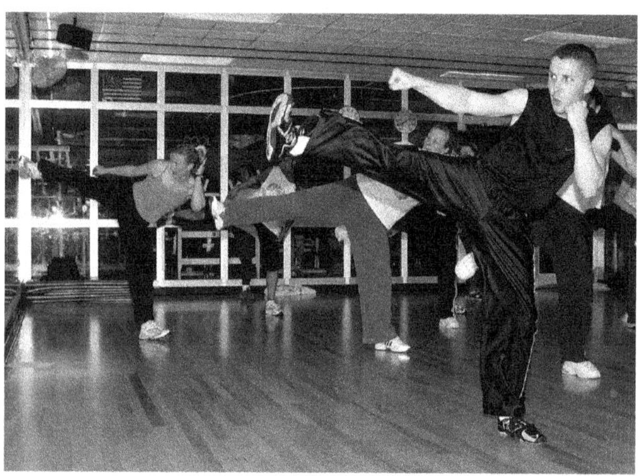

**Types of Physical Fitness:**

Consider fitness for a moment. When we talk about becoming more physically fit, what does that really mean? What is physical fitness? There are three types or three areas of physical fitness.

**Cardiovascular Fitness**

Cardiovascular fitness means that we have a strong, healthy heart. The heart is nothing more than a muscle. Like other muscles, it must be used and exercised to stay healthy. Eating a low fat, low cholesterol diet helps to prevent cholesterol buildup in our arteries. If we eat too much saturated fat or cholesterol, then plaque will build up in our arteries. This plaque buildup is called arteriosclerosis. The result of plaque buildup is that our arteries become like a clogged pipe. This makes our heart have to work harder. Clogged arteries also are less flexible and can make us more prone towards suffering from strokes.

A stroke is when an artery bursts from too much blood pressure and lack of flexibility in the walls of the artery because they are hardened with plaque. Maintaining a low level of sodium in our diet can help reduce the chances of high blood pressure. Exercise can help flex the arteries and keep them soft and flexible, thus reducing the chances of stroke. Exercise also causes the release of certain chemicals within our body which have the effect of helping to "flush" cholesterol out of the blood stream and minimize the buildup of plaque on the walls of our arteries.

The disadvantage of developing fat is that it can also cause our heart to work harder all of the time. As fat cells grow in size, the veins and arteries between these cells grow in length. This makes our circulatory system larger so that we have more "pipes", but we still have the same size of "pump"; the heart. The end result is that the heart is working much harder than it needs to to keep the blood flowing even when we are not exercising.

When an overweight person does exercise, they are making even greater demands upon their heart. That is why all exercise programs should be undertaken on a gradual basis. Start slowly, with very light exercise and build up to more advanced levels as your weight drops and you develop more stamina and cardiovascular strength.

Having cardiovascular fitness means maintaining a diet low in sodium, cholesterol and saturated fat, getting enough exercise to keep our blood vessels flexible, work the heart muscle and "flush" cholesterol out of our system.

If our fitness goal is to develop better cardiovascular fitness, then we need to look at our diet and what levels of cholesterol, sodium and saturated fat we are consuming on a regular basis. These components of our diet must be reduced. We must engage in physical activities which will gradually build our heart strength. Walking, biking, swimming, rowing, jogging in very moderate amounts and at very moderate rates are all excellent ways to begin developing cardiovascular fitness.

These are all aerobic exercises. They should be done at least three times per week for periods of 20-30 minutes. Jogging for 5 minutes or biking for 10 minutes does not develop cardiovascular fitness. If anything, it is more of a strain on the heart than a benefit. 20-30 minutes gives the heart a chance to get up to speed, maintain a good level of muscular activity for a reasonable amount of time and then slow down and return to a normal rate.

All the while you are exercising and training to get into better shape, your body is "tuning" itself to use oxygen more efficiently. For every breath that you take, your body is getting more mileage out of the oxygen that you are consuming.

## Flexibility

Fitness goals are not necessarily accomplished independently of each other. While we are improving our cardiovascular fitness, we may also be working on the next area of fitness, flexibility. As mentioned earlier, our arteries gain flexibility through exercise. Our muscles also gain flexibility through exercise. Flexibility is another measure of physical fitness. If we do not have flexibility, then we are not totally physically fit.

There are many stretches and exercises than we can perform to increase our flexibility. Flexibility is very important because, tight, inflexible muscles, tendons, and joints can restrict our movement and do not give us adequate support for our daily activities. A body that has little flexibility is more prone towards injury.

## Muscular Flexibility

There are two types of flexibility, muscular flexibility and joint flexibility. Muscular flexibility is concerned with the muscles, tendons and ligaments. To increase our muscular flexibility we must stretch - more on stretching in a bit.

**Joint Flexibility**

In addition to flexibility in our muscles, tendons and ligaments, we must develop flexibility in our joints. Theses goals are not just for athletes or martial artists alone. Good physical fitness and flexibility should be everyone's goal for life. You're never too old to begin or to keep going. Just remember to build your training in small increments. That is the way to prevent injury and insure maximum benefit. Joint flexibility allows more freedom of movement of the joint, less pain and stiffness and less chance of injury or damage to the joint.

**Strength**

Strength is the third area of physical fitness. It does little good to have excellent cardiovascular health, great flexibility and little or no strength. Strength does not mean lifting weights to become an internationally recognized body builder. Strength means increasing your amount of muscle mass. The more muscle mass that you have, the more control that you can have over your body and its movements. Good muscle strength makes it possible to get a better workout and develop more cardiovascular fitness. If you have very little muscle, your muscles may get worn out quickly and prevent you from continuing in a workout.

If strength is part of your fitness goals, then you will be focusing on physical activities that will gradually build your strength in different ways. Biking is excellent for the legs. Moderate weight lifting in a supervised program is excellent for overall strength development. Swimming is excellent for working all of the muscles in the body. It does not build very large muscle mass, but it does increase the strength and endurance of the existing muscles. Martial arts helps build legs, arms and chest, back and stomach muscles and most other muscle groups.

To meet your strength development goals you should identify exercises and activities that will work the muscle groups that you seek to develop. Also make sure that these exercises will help develop the muscles to the extent that you would like. Not all exercises will build large muscle mass, but they will improve muscle condition, tone and flexibility. Lastly, it is not necessary to gain huge muscle mass and muscle density, but it is beneficial to increase it if that is a deficiency of yours so that your strength increases above your current levels to make you more fit in this area.

## *Planning Your Fitness Program*

The earlier section on *Goal Setting* tells us to identify our goals and develop a plan to meet them. In the case of physical fitness goals, we have the three areas of physical fitness cardiovascular fitness, flexibility and strength. A good balance between all three should be achieved and maintained for good overall physical fitness. Below are some general tips to consider when planning and engaging in a physical fitness program.

### Fitness Training Program Planning Tips

1. Identify which areas need improvement.
2. Write down the specific goals that you intend to accomplish in each area.
3. Identify exercises or activities that will support these goals.
4. Develop a realistic training schedule.
5. Keep your log book and measure your progress.
6. Reevaluate your progress often to see if any adjustments need to be made to your goals, time frame for reaching them or your training schedule.

## *Sports Training and Physical Conditioning Tips*

Sports training and martial arts training should be undertaken with the idea that there are no overnight wonders. The best way to make progress in martial arts or any other training is to train consistently over a long period of time. This approach to training helps the individual develop discipline in the training regimen and good conditioning habits.

There is no benefit in training every day for a solid month, only to miss several weeks, then returning to training everyday and missing more time. The instructors suggest that you train twice a week consistently. With a schedule of twice per week students should be able to maintain their martial arts training even if other activities are making demands upon their schedule. If possible three times per week is ideal.

**Perfect Practice Makes Perfect**

The old saying about practice makes perfect should be rewritten to say that perfect practice makes perfect. There is no point in practicing over and over if you are doing the wrong moves or practicing bad techniques. The only way that progress can be made is to know what the correct moves or techniques are and the correct method of executing them. Then you must practice with intensity. Whenever you have a question about proper technique or the correct moves ask your instructors.

Remember, when you are practicing for either tournaments or self defense situations, the way that you practice is the way that you will perform. Aside from developing and emphasizing bad technique or incorrect moves, incorrect practice could result in injuries such as strained knees or other undesirable conditions such as pulled muscles.

Like all sports and physical activities, martial arts are not without occasional injuries and minor setbacks. Martial artists, like other athletes, often experience sore muscles, minor sprains and aches. You will notice that the more consistently that you train without long periods of inactivity, the better your conditioning will be and the less likely it is that you will experience minor injuries such as pulled muscles. Think about your body like a fine-tuned high performance race car. Without the proper treatment, maintenance and care you will not get the optimal performance that you seek.

**Stretching**

Stretching helps reduce injuries, increase speed of motion, range of motion, general mobility and improve coordination.

There are two types of stretching: stretching to increase flexibility and stretching to increase mobility. When beginning a workout I have students loosen up very lightly before starting so that they can carefully work out any muscle and joint stiffness that they may have when they come into the dojo. It is critical for students to loosen up before exercising. Stretching helps increase mobility of muscles and joints in preparation for the exercises, drills and other workout content to which students will be subjected. You should do incremental stretching throughout the workout or training session.

Joints and muscles that are more fluid are not as susceptible to injury and can help the martial artist with increased speed in his techniques. This benefit is both physical and psychological. For example, I know that when certain muscles or joints are tight or stiff, I will not move as quickly and I will have a conscious aversion to moving a joint or muscle as quickly as I know that I could otherwise, simply because I am aware of the reduced mobility and the possibility that it will cause damage.

The improved coordination of flexible muscles and joints comes from the greater control and fluidity that result from effective stretching. Muscles and joints that are more fluid and mobile are easier to control and allow the martial artist to more easily practice drills that aid in coordination and agility. Improved speed comes from having generally looser joints and muscles so that reactions and direct actions can be carried out without the negative resistance caused by less resilient muscles and joints. Flexibility also aids in a greater balance among the various muscles and more fluid, less choppy, wasteful movement and conservation of energy.

Stretch every day, even if you are not coming to class on a given day. Stretching helps maintain the flexibility that you have gained in your training. The stretching that we do in class is mainly designed just to loosen you up for the class session. At home or in the Dojang before or after class is where you should really concentrate on developing flexibility on your own.

Stretching should definitely be done for at least a few minutes after each class. This is the time that you are most warmed up and your muscles, tendons and ligaments are most pliable and responsive to careful stretching. Stretching should be a relaxing activity. We can do as many pushups or other exercises as we might want and do them as fast as we want, but when it comes to stretching, that is the time to slow down and take your time.

Stretching should always be done carefully and slowly. Never bob or bounce while you stretch. It is easy to strain or pull a muscle while bouncing during a stretch. Stretch gently. Muscles must expand and contract slowly. If you pull a muscle, you must avoid stretching or training until the muscle has had time to repair itself. Follow the recommendations for treating minor sports injuries in the section of that name.

If you stretch too far, but you do not pull a muscle, you may be quite sore for the next day or two. This means that you may have torn some muscle tissue and you must give that tissue time to heal. When a tear or pull occurs, your muscles will form scar tissue. That is why you should not workout if you have pulled a muscle, even if only slightly.

**The Workout**

Working out hard every day is not recommended because usually during hard workouts you will cause a normal amount of tissue scarring. This is what builds larger, stronger muscles. That is why weight lifters increase the size of their muscles. As they lift weight or work the muscles, the muscles experience small tears. For the next 24 to 48 hours these tears will heal and the muscle tissue reinforces itself, making it stronger and larger.

If you do not train for more than a few days or a week, this extra tissue immediately begins to break down and the muscle starts to loose size and flexibility. That is why you should make every attempt to train regularly and consistently, even if only twice per week. This will provide you with the best results and conditioning.

**Warming Up**

Warm up slowly. This gives the body, joints, muscles, tendons, heart and arteries time to warm up because of the increased blood flow through them. Let your system gradually adjust to the new level of activity. As the blood flow increase through the muscles and joints, they will become more flexible.

After warming up it may be a good idea to do some light stretching for a few minutes before getting into the main part of the workout where you will be doing physical activity for an extended period of time (20-30 minutes). This stretching will make you loose enough to perform the main part of the workout while reducing the chances of a strain or pulled muscle.

**Maintaining the Pace**

The main part of the workout is where you are either increasing your aerobic stamina or your muscle strength. Flexibility is developed after the workout.

Increasing your aerobic stamina is done by maintaining a consistent level of physical activity where your heart is beating at what is called the Target Heart Rate. The minimum amount of time required to develop cardiovascular fitness or aerobic stamina is 20-30 minutes, three times per week. The heart must beat consistently in the target range (explained below) in order for the heart to receive an adequate workout or exercise. Remember it is a muscle too and you are trying to develop its fitness.

## Target Heart Rate

The normal resting heart beat ranges from 70 for most people to about 40 for more fit people. Less effort is required from a healthy heart to supply oxygen to the body than from an unconditioned heart. As you age, your target heart rate range gradually gets lower. Children and young adults have higher target heart rates than older adults and middle aged adults. You can look online for any number of target rate calculators. Then consider wearing a heart rate monitor to make sure you stay within your range. Going too high can be dangerous and not getting your heart rate high enough will prevent you from obtaining the full benefit of your workout.

## Cooling Down

After the main part of the workout is complete, you should spend anywhere from 2-5 minutes cooling down. Cooling down does not mean simply stopping and having something cold to drink. This is the time that you do several easy, low intensity exercises designed to keep you moving and allow your heart rate to come down out of the target range to a rate slightly above the normal resting rate. You are gradually bringing yourself to a stop.

After several minutes of cool-down, you can then stop without causing a shock or strain to your system. Then you are ready to enter the flexibility phase of the workout.

## Developing Flexibility

Flexibility is developed best when the muscles are warm. Muscles are more pliable and supple right after the workout and the cool down. Once your heart has just about returned to its normal resting rate from finishing the cool-down, you can begin stretching.

The stretching that you do after the warm-up is simply loosening up to prevent injury and to allow your muscles and joints to move freely enough during the main workout to prevent injury. The initial loosening up does not increase your overall flexibility.

Now your goal is to increase your level of flexibility in specific areas. Stretching should be done slowly, gradually and carefully. Never force muscles or joints to work harder than is comfortable. The old saying "No pain, no gain" is false. Take your time and develop your flexibility slowly.

**Practicing Forms (Kata – Japanese/Okinawan, Hyungs or Poomse in Korean)**

There are numerous benefits to practicing forms. In order to achieve these benefits, the forms must be practiced in the correct way.

## Tips for Practicing Forms

1. Learn all of the moves correctly.
2. Understand the practical application and meaning of each move.
3. Practice each move with power.
4. Practice the form with a constant rhythm or tempo.
5. Concentrate on controlling and pacing your breathing. One recommended approach is to exhale as you do each move. This will cause you to automatically inhale before you do the next move. By keeping your breathing regulated you will not become dizzy or light-headed and your moves will have more power. Breathing controls endurance.
6. Know the meaning of the forms.
7. Practice all of your forms. This will help to improve your technique and you will discover ways to improve your overall power, speed and coordination. As you improve your performance of forms your mind and body begin to function together. Movement and control become intuitive. Soon, you will not consciously think about movement. You will simply react.
8. Forms should be practiced with intensity. A form is an ancient way of pretending to defend yourself against multiple attackers from different directions. The more effective you become at forms and controlling your movements, the better you will become at fighting in tournaments or in a self-defense situation because you have developed the ability to intuitively move in many directions rapidly and efficiently without wasting time or energy. Forms should be practiced with fierce intensity as if you are actually defending yourself.
9. Practice a form five times in a row. This helps you to learn the pattern of the movements. This helps the student retain in their memory the basic pattern so that it will flow in their mind.
10. Practice the form at the correct speed with attention to balance. Good balance is essential for solid technique. Pay particular attention to your balance as you change from stance to stance. Your posture should be alert, energized, strong -Don't just move, feel the form.

11. Practice the foam as fast as possible. This is another memory aid. If you can fly through a form, then you know the pattern of the moves.
12. Practice the form very slowly, one move at a time. Take the first move and study yourself. Make sure that your hands, feet, head, shoulders etc. are correctly positioned. Make a mental note of the details. If you have learned the correct positioning for each move, then you will know what to look for to critique yourself. Do this for every move in the form. Then go through the form again and try to correct the details. Every time you practice, correct the imperfections and improve your technique.

Learning the moves in a form is like learning the letters of the alphabet. After you have learned the letters, you can begin to read and write. Learning the forms on several levels means that you will learn how to relate your movements to those of another person when you are sparring. You will begin to understand the nature of change, redirection of force, the feeling of dynamic balance and the difference between hard and soft. During forms your body and muscles are constantly fluctuating between relaxed looseness and a taught explosive release of power.

Forms benefit internal and external muscles. The muscles of the arms and legs are strengthened as well as the internal muscles such as those inside the abdomen or the other internal muscles supporting internal organs. No other physical activity develops every single muscle group in the way the martial arts forms do. Forms require your body to move in every possible direction that it can go. Forms also require total mental concentration. Becoming more effective at forms improves the student's ability to clear his or her mind of extraneous thoughts.

At some point, the ultimate purpose of forms is to develop your skill, balance, timing and coordination. No one will ever defend themselves on the street by deciding to execute their green-belt form any more than a musician would go perform a C-major scale for a concert. Forms are exercises, in a real self-defense situation, movement will need to be spontaneous and free flowing; a mixing of many movements as appropriate for the situation. What is important is to learn the Bunkai or interpretation of the movements. Each movement in a form has one or more potential combat applications. That is why they were developed. Unfortunately, this knowledge is typically lost on most instructors and what many schools will teach is "B" knowledge as a quick route to providing some "plausible" explanation that has no practical basis in reality.

Learning practical applications for realistic scenarios is a time investment that is well worth it, but not typically part of the curriculum of most schools; therefore forms are generally reduced to mere exercise and treated as an academic requirement for advancement to the next level. Many schools will include additional self-defense techniques in their curriculum as a substitute for teaching a practical application of the movement in the forms. This often serves to confuse students more as they can easily conclude that the self-defense techniques may have a practical use, the sparring certainly adds realism, fun and great workout and that leaves forms as some required element of the curriculum that has no apparent real benefit other than memorization and condition.

An excellent book on the entire subject of Bunkai is "**The Way of Kata**" by Lawrence Kane. It takes movements common to many martial arts styles and explains several possible practical interpretations of those movements. Once you begin to practice each movement separately as you would your "street self-defense" techniques, you begin to see that they are practical and lethal and deserve serious study to increase you martial skills. Once that door of knowledge and discovery is opened, students rarely question the utility of studying and practicing forms.

## *Coordination*

Coordination is a skill you must develop just like many other qualities. You are born with a certain amount of coordination for your particular body. You must work to maintain and improve this. Coordination is the ability to make the body do what the mind requires.

Visualization helps coordination. Picture what you are trying to do. If you cannot picture it, it will be more difficult to accomplish. Therefore, coordination consists of mating the mind's vision with the body's ability. Many different things may affect your level of coordination positively or negatively; timing, speed, balance and flexibility are just a few.

As you practice coordination with different drills, you will see that it becomes easier to adapt to new techniques and training methods. Adaptability in martial arts is key to survival. As you improve at adapting, you will become more coordinated. The other part of coordination is distance judgment. If you reach too far or not far enough because you have misjudged the distance, then you will need to practice distance improvement. This will aid your coordination.

One of the best ways to improve coordination is simply to drill your various kicks, punches and other technique endlessly with stationary and moving targets and at different distances and speeds. What happens over time is that your body becomes programmed and develops the necessary muscle memory and improved technique so that you move more gracefully and confidently.

I have seen many students, particularly adults, come in at the start of the martial arts training. They can barely put one foot in front of the other and walk without tripping on themselves. After a few short months of training in different stances and working through the movements in the kata, they are able move with ease because their muscles had never really been taught to do anything requiring any degree of coordination. They realized that coordination is not something you are born with, but like balance, it is a skill that must be developed.

## Balance

Balance in movement and posture means that you should be able to smoothly, shift weight or adjust muscles that are supporting you and your position. When trying to deceive an opponent you will need to develop the ability to cause this shift in balance invisibly and imperceptibly so that your opponent will not notice and then you will have the advantage.

To move, stand, sit, kick or punch in a jerky, awkward way is not to have balance. Real balance means knowing when, where and how much to move to stay in this position without thinking about it. Know what to do without thinking. If you must think about it, you do not have balance, because you cannot think of balance and fight at the same time. If you do not have balance, you cannot fight.

The variety of drills, kata movements and conditioning techniques will improve your balance and coordination very quickly. These improved physical qualities along with your improving strength, flexibility and endurance begin to combine to transform your body into an effective fighting platform.

## Relaxation

Relaxation is one of the first and most difficult lessons that the martial artist must learn. You cannot really be taught how to relax; it must be discovered and practiced. There are certainly tips you can follow as to certain activities that can bring about a sense of relaxation or get you in a mental state where you can begin to relax yourself, but for the most part, relaxation is something you have to begin to find yourself and sense like a mental state you seeking.

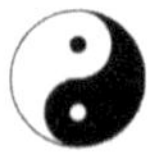

To be relaxed is to be prepared to perceive. Perception is critical. In martial arts and in any aspect of your life, perception enables you to pick up on details you might not have noticed. It enables you to sense your environment, which can be used as an aid in your own defense or survival and it enables you to sense your opponent or your own physical condition and limits at any given moment. When a martial artist is able to perceive his opponent's intentions without a bad attitude or anger or other distractions of the moment, then the martial artist is mentally capable of using some strategy or tactic to counter them.

To be in a state other than relaxation such as tension and distraction is to be affected by other things or thoughts and to not be capable of full awareness that enables you to perceive things that are essential.

## *Meditation*

Martial artists borrow tradition from various Asian warrior monks. Monks practice meditation for religious contemplation. Meditation by martial artists is not for religious fulfillment, but for contemplation, focus and channeling of Chi and enlightenment. You can use meditation for several purposes, to solve a problem, to empty the mind, to find an answer, to discover harmony, direction, organization, peace and to embrace the enlightenment. The sun is the light force in our solar system. It emanates its positive energy to the planets and the energy transfers to them and is absorbed; and it gives life. The absence of this light takes life away.

A martial artist meditates to empty the mind and the ego before a training session. He or she must empty the cup of their emotions, thoughts and desires and prepare the mind, body and spirit. You must align the Chi (the energy force) of the body positively to prepare to absorb new knowledge and to reach higher levels of understanding, insight and attainment of skill in the course of your workout.

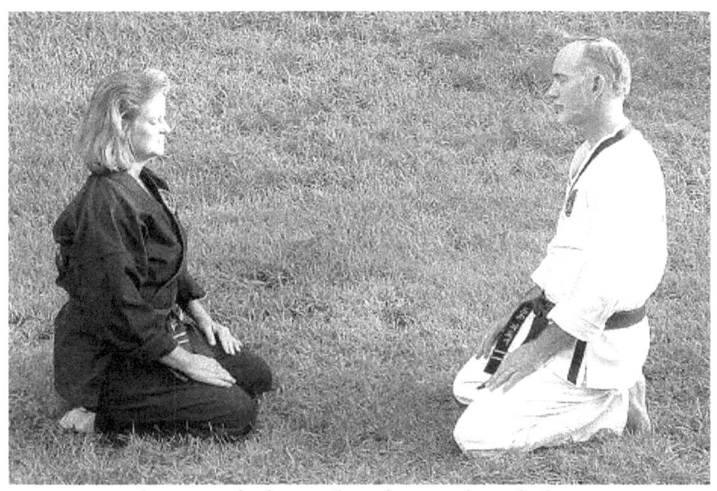

*Meditation helps calm the soul and sharpen your focus for learning*

Meditate and focus on light. Focus on a conscious awareness of your thoughts. What are the positive thoughts and what are your negative thoughts? Focus on the positive thoughts. Replace negative perspectives and energy with positive. Change your thoughts from negative to positive. This is preparation for experiencing a more effective, productive and positive training session. This is a preparation for a more positive outcome to relationships and events in your life.

Change your thoughts and you will change your actions, your outcomes and thus the reactions of others to you. Negative thoughts will attempt to creep in and you must expend energy to deflect them and replace them as they attempt to interrupt your positive cycle. Pay attention to the positives and ignore, forget or replace the negatives and your internal energy will begin to cycle in a positive direction and negative cycles will be reversed. You will begin to emanate positive rather than negative energy. Focus your Chi on each moment of each day, of each person, of each situation. Pay attention and change each thought and action in a conscious way. In Zen, it is eating when you eat and sleeping when you sleep.

Be where you are. Organize your attention on the situation at hand. This organization is positive, the disorganization of not paying attention and not focusing yourself on the situation is negative energy and yields negative results. Stress, negativity and discord begin to replace positive Chi when you interrupt your focus.

Many of us feel stress because our body is in one place while our mind and focus is elsewhere. This phenomenon separates mind from body. It interrupts your spirit and disrupts any positive Chi you might have been experiencing. Meditation prepares you to unite mind and body.

The whole notion of multi-tasking in today's modern age is an interruption of focus and a separation of mind and body from the same task. The result is that you perform no task well. The human can only perform one physical task at a time and that task requires mental oversight. If the mind is elsewhere while the body is attempting to perform a task then the task will not be effective or successful. When the mind attempts to perform two or more tasks, it cannot perform them in parallel.

Consciously we can only manage one task in one instant. We delude ourselves into thinking that we can multi-task, when all we are doing is one task at a time. We are lining tasks up one after the other, or worse, we attempt a portion of one for an instant, then a portion of another, for another instant or two, then back to the first, then the second, then possibly adding on a third. If any one of these tasks requires some degree of extended concentration beyond a stolen instant or two that task is in danger of failing and generally will. Likewise, the body begins to fatigue and become stressed due to the separation from mind in these ill-fated attempts to multi-task. As the monks instruct, eat when you eat, walk when you walk.

The spirit is most at peace when the mind and body are connected working in harmony and in the same place at the same time. Try this and you will see that the positive energy expended to maintain focus yields positive energy. The negative energy generated as you allow your focus to shift elsewhere yields negative energy around you.

Your meditation should focus on conscious identification of what positive and negative roles you play in the lives of those around you. Replace the negative ones, visualize the positive roles that you do or will play. Meditate to visualize the martial skills that you seek. Visualize, in your mind's eye, yourself performing techniques the way you wish to perform them. Prior to starting your meditation it is useful to set a goal for your meditation; pick a subject you wish to contemplate and focus entirely on it, purging other thoughts.

## *Energy*

Train so that you are always ready. Eat well so that you will be generally healthy, but be able and ready to fight without having eaten or prepared. That is the nature of truly being ready for self-defense or any type of combat.

Food and vitamins are essential to proper functioning of the body, but be able to function well at all times and do not focus on hunger, pain, discomforts of climate, other distractions or fatigue. You must be able to go on even with these annoyances and distractions. Your survival may depend upon it.

Energy is a precious resource of the body. You must be conservative with it. In a prolonged encounter, you will need all you can muster. A novice or intermediate student will be brimming with energy and adrenalin. They are excited or apprehensive about sparring or having an encounter. We all are. The difference is that the more advanced student learns control. Discipline yourself to relax so that you will not burn vital energy and tire quickly. Then the energy will be available when you need a quick burst in a dramatic moment. When you are relaxed, you will burn less energy and be able to focus more effectively. Combat requires short periods of intense action and this demands considerable energy.

## *Martial Exercises vs. Traditional Calisthenics*

Most martial arts schools begin their training classes with a warm up period containing traditional calisthenics; jumping jacks, push ups, jogging in place and the like. As I discussed earlier, this exercises are all part of increasing your strength, stamina and flexibility. My approach to warming up a class is that everything you do should have some martial application.

The exercises you perform should have some basis in the types of movements you will likely execute in a real self-defense situation. You are studying martial arts and the goal of improving your skill is to increase your odds of survival on the street or wherever you happen to be. When I have a group conduct warm-ups, they are practicing for survival, even in a fun way. Here are a few examples of how cardio vascular, strengthening and conditioning exercises can be accomplished in a more combat-realistic setting:

Rather than do push-ups, I have students do punch push-ups. Each time the student comes up in the push-up, they throw a punch forward toward an opponent who may be on the ground with them.

Rather than do jumping jacks, I have students to punching jacks where they throw a punch on each landing while holding their hands in a boxing position ready to defend themselves.

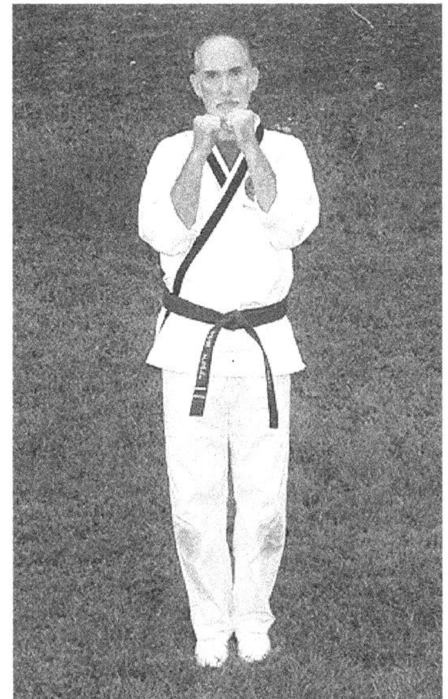
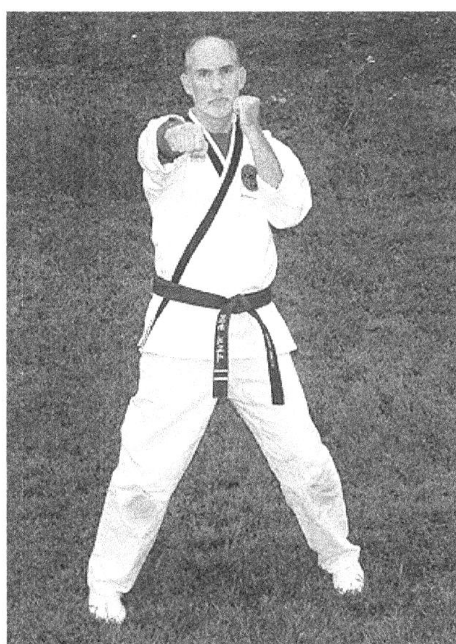

*Punching jacks*

I have students simply crawl on their belly from one end of the dojo to the other and back. Sometimes we string lines of rope the length of the dojo and tell them that their head must stay low so that it does not touch the rope. These drills teach them a practical skill if they had to sneak away from an assailant, crawl under a truck or other object for cover from someone searching for them or simply crawl down a smoke-filled hallway in a burning building. If they get used to crawling in practice then they will not be so disoriented by the idea that they might need to do so in real life. It will seem like a natural option for survival.

Below is a drill consisting of ground sidekicks. The student does a sidekick then switches hands and turns the body to the other side to execute a sidekick with the opposite leg. This is continued back and forth.

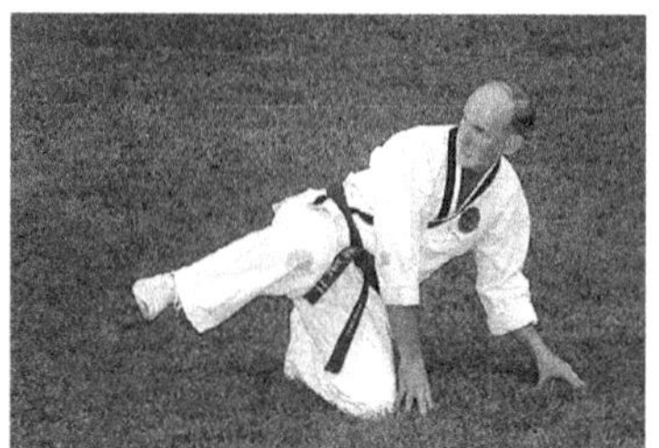
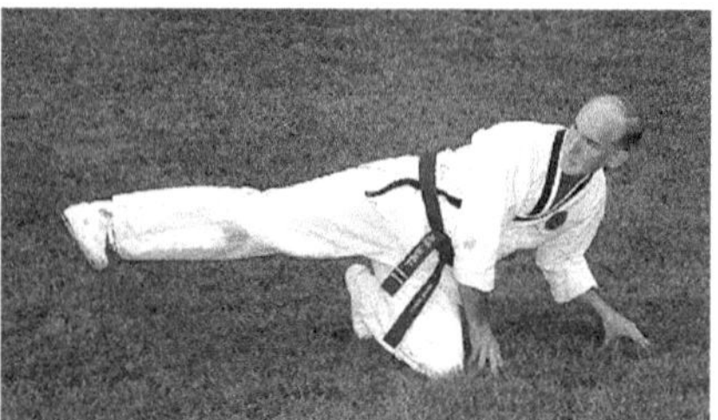

*Ground sidekicks*

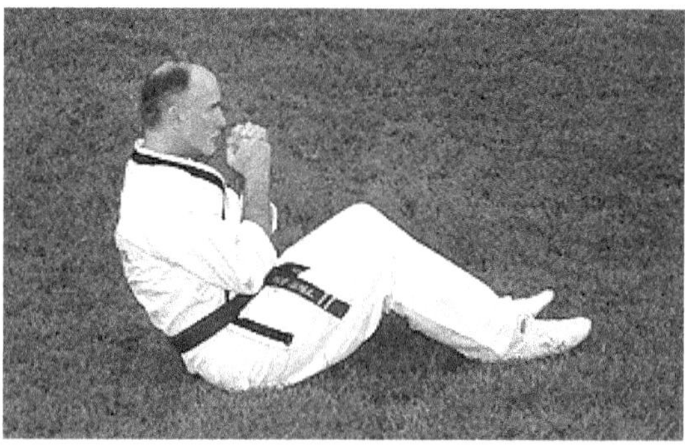

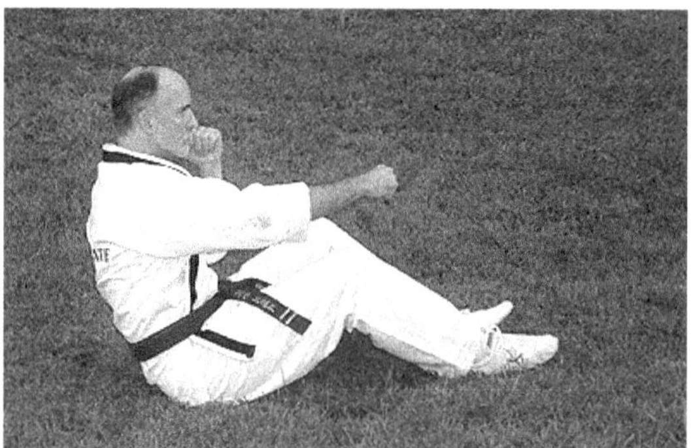

*Punch sit-ups*

Rather than only doing various types of sit-ups, I have students do punch sit-ups. They either rise up and fire two-punches straight ahead, or they rise up and fire a right punch to the left and a left punch to the right. The idea is that the student is ready and able and trained to be prepared to fight from any position. Doing workout drills with more of a martial flair to them gives the drills more significance than simply saying that sit-ups are to build strong abdominal muscles and nothing else. Another variation on the punch sit-ups is to roll quickly to one side, then sit-up and punch. The roll is an escape from your opponent by quickly moving to the side.

Often when students are doing the "crawl for life" we will have instructors or other students hitting them with padded bats and throwing various relatively safe objects at them such as training pads. This creates a more distracting and hostile environment while they are trying to crawl, keep their head down and now keep their head covered to protect it from injuries by objects or assailants.

Many of these drills are classroom versions of military obstacle courses and are intended to serve the same purpose; to prepare the student for combat and for unpleasant situations. These few examples give you the idea of how traditional calisthenics are replaced with similar exercises with the same physical benefits, but with an added component of practical survival skill building built in.

## *Building Your Library of Techniques*

When you are comfortable with certain techniques, stop using them for a while and work to become comfortable with several others. This change of focus helps build your repertoire.

When training, work on what does not come naturally until it becomes natural, then work on something new. It does not develop your skill to spend time on techniques that you have mastered. Remember the techniques that you have mastered were once unnatural and required practice.

Never be comfortable with where you are. There is always more skill or knowledge to acquire. If you think there is no more knowledge or skill to acquire, and then reflect on this. Study others and you will see that you have much that you can learn and do. There is no end to it.

## *Injuries and Healing*

In a real fight, try not to ever let your opponent see that you are injured. Play off your injury if possible. Even if your injury is visible or noticeable, let your opponent think that it is not affecting you. This will make him stop and think that maybe his techniques are ineffective. In other situations, depending upon the opponent and the circumstances you may want to pretend that you are injured worse than you are – this is using a martial arts concept known as the strategies of opposites. Pretending to have a more serious injury can give your opponent a false sense of security by thinking that he is close to defeating you. Then you will have him. This is deception at its best.

It also helps not to focus on you. Keep your eyes and your mind on your opponent in a real fight. Injuries can be dealt with later; a real opponent must be dealt with immediately. Even if you have been stabbed with a knife or shot once or even twice, people do not always die from a single gunshot wound or knife stab. You can continue to function, but you must focus, not on the pain or the shock of the injury, but on surviving. Your will to survive and your ability to focus are the two primary factors in determining your ultimate survival.

If you are training and you receive an injury, tend to it immediately. Prolonging the treatment could make it worse. Do not make a big deal of the injury every time or you will be easily distracted in a real fight. Learn to be able to tell what is serious and what is minor, but do take care of it.

Do not train with injuries that could worsen by training. Allow the injury time to heal completely, and then slowly work back into your routine with caution.

## Limits

Everything and everyone has limits. Know what they are. This may be the limit of someone's patience or your own. You need to know the limit or length of your kicks. You need to know your physical limits of endurance or strength or speed.

Every time you train or if you are in the midst of a self-defense situation, make a note and pay attention to your physical and mental limits. If you know that you cannot lift a certain weight or run a certain distance, then do not do it. If you have a current limit, you can however, gradually, slowly and with care, extend this limit. Begin sparring for one minute. Do this for as long as it takes until one minute is no longer a challenge or a benefit, then increase to one and a half minutes and so on until you are working for good lengths of time.

Know your mental limits as well. If you cannot develop or gather the ideas for some strategy of defense then consider what weakness you may need to address that will increase your understanding or make it possible for you to develop the strategy that you would like. There is a gap in your knowledge, skill, training or experience. Figure out what is missing and address it. Read more books, speak with more instructors, hit the internet for information, change your training. When you discover the gap, address it, work to fill it and eventually your weakness in that area will improve.

Back up from the problem or the challenge and take one piece at a time, this makes everything easier. Once you reassemble all of the pieces, you will be able to define your limit and extend it because you understand why it is a limit and why it is holding you back.

## *Frustration*

Why do you get frustrated? If you understood what caused you to be frustrated in your training, maybe you would not be frustrated. Like an injury, do not dwell on it or focus on the fact you're frustrated or you will become distracted. Realize that you have reached a point of frustration, figure out why and focus on improving or changing what is causing the frustration. Frustration also stems from either not knowing your limits or simply not being willing or patient enough with yourself to accept your current limits and work within them.

Be realistic. Progress comes from pushing yourself to a degree, but do it in a realistic and achievable manner. Trying to run a marathon without training for it and becoming frustrated when you are exhausted after the first half-mile is a case of setting yourself up for failure because you have not properly trained for such a goal. Some frustration can be avoided by taking a realistic assessment of what your abilities and limits are and working from that point of reality forward as opposed to simply deciding what you would like to eventually do and then jumping directly into it. Preparation is the key to success. If you fail to plan, then you have just created a plan to fail.

Frustration can be an obstacle or deterrent or a temporary roadblock to further progress. Frustration is an emotion that masks another problem and if focused on can cause a temporary or even permanent mental sense of defeat. Many people decide in a moment of frustration and emotion to throw in the towel. They have now defeated themselves. Change your focus and fix the problem. The emotion associated with frustration prevents progress and learning. Therefore, it is important to understand the kinds of things that can cause frustration so that you may address them or prevent them by adequate planning and preparation for new challenges.

You may become frustrated when your instructor explains something; you try it and you are not successful because you did not understand the explanation. If you failed to understand the explanation, that is the instructor's fault, not yours. Ask your instructor to explain it until you understand better what you are attempting to learn. Ask your instructor or ask yourself what you should do to prepare better physically or mentally for a new challenge. Once you have addressed this, then you can proceed with the lesson, better equipped for success.

You may be frustrated by the complexity of something new that you are learning. If it is too complex to take in at once, break it down into manageable steps. This is so simple, but very few people practice this. You must approach anything new, difficult or challenging by dividing it. You have heard the saying divide and conquer. Why take on the entirety of a problem, when you can solve it in pieces. Try it. This will remove much frustration. You will see that nearly anything is doable if broken down into small enough pieces. There is no secret here, only work, willingness and persistence.

You cannot become a black belt or a highly skilled martial artist overnight. Everyone knows this. You must build your black belt skill and knowledge over years of carefully structured learning and training. It's a rewarding and exciting journey – enjoy the trip!

## *Respect*

Respect for someone or their achievements or position is an important part of a cohesive society. Respect is often the most important and the first lesson of the martial arts. Respect means to have a high opinion or to hold someone in high esteem. Respect is the ability to appreciate the significance, the value and the importance of a person, their character or their achievements. My wife and I often emphasize to our children the need to respect other's property or to respect something that was given as a gift –

no matter how small or inexpensive. Hold that gift in esteem as a symbol of affection from the giver. This shows respect for the person who gave the gift.

Respect must be developed and maintained by the student. It is a process of learning what is of value and worth and then making note of it and keeping that significance always in mind. Respect aids self-discipline, which is essential to development and learning.

Respect is also the beginning of developing an open mind. Part of being open minded is respecting others ideas, people and styles without respect, very little is possible. However, it is easy to respect something or someone with which you agree. The challenge comes in trying to respect someone or something with which you do not agree. It is important to hold someone else's opinions and position in high regard because they do. It is all part of respecting that individual even if you do not hold the same opinions. This allows for more civil behavior and relationships between people of different backgrounds and opinions. Respect other people and opinions without subjugating your own or allowing theirs to co-opt yours. In the end, you may not actually hold someone in high-regard where you feel that you can actually respect them, and they may not be worthy of respect, but you can at least be civil toward them.

## *Etiquette*

A martial artist is strong in character, personality and confidence. Fighting skill and strategy is assumed. Etiquette should be expected at any level.

Those who are high in skill, rank or experience should practice etiquette or courtesy and politeness with those who are less experienced and the converse as well. Etiquette and courtesy is a sign of self-confidence, strength and security, not a sign of weakness or submissiveness. The basis of etiquette is respect. Understand this well. All martial artists should practice this.

In the days of the Samurai and even in medieval Europe, warriors and knights faced each other in mass or single combat, but they held a certain professional respect for each other; understanding that the skill of their opponents was acquired through much hard work, discipline, sacrifice and dedication. While two opponents or opposing forces might be enemies, their common ideals and traits as warriors engendered a mutual respect.

## *Ego*

Guard your ego most carefully. It is a two-edged sword. Ego manifests itself as emotion. Emotions that are negative such as anger or hate will blind you when you are in the midst of battle or anywhere.

If ego becomes negative, emotions including fear, anger or hate will keep one from having an open mind. Without an open mind, the student of martial arts will wither and die from lack of new knowledge, thought and experiences.

A good fighter must be a good thinker and a good thinker only becomes that way by developing an open mind to others and their ideas. Learn from and respect all others. Consider everything and you will grow in skill and knowledge.

Ego that manifests itself as positive emotion; self-confidence, pride, self-realization is a great thing. It is the key to building confidence and self-assuredness. A positive ego can give a fighter the conviction to overcome his or her own insecurity, doubt or fear of a superior opponent.

You must guard a positive ego as well as a negative ego. Do not be blatant or over-indulgent in a positive ego or you may disorient those around you. This is again, where balance is important. Develop balance and strength in these areas. A healthy ego means you possess enough self-confidence that you do not feel the need to over-assert your ego at the risk of offending those around you.

## *Keeping an Open Mind*

Have an open mind to new styles, techniques and opinions of others. These things are not a threat. An open mind is strength and a security and enables you to become more skilled, competent and valuable in martial arts, school, work and in life. A closed mind to new ideas will make them a greater threat because you will not benefit from what new people or ideas have to offer and they will be ahead of you in these areas. An open mind is never bad because it develops awareness and awareness is essential to survival anywhere. When the mind is closed, it is unaware. When the mind is unaware, it is at risk.

## *Martial Arts as Art Form*

What are Karate, Kung Fu, Kendo or the other many styles? They are fighting arts; means of self-defense. However, we often forget in our training that they are most definitely art forms; the art of self-defense. An art form is a means of expression through some medium. For the painter, his medium may be oil paint on canvas or the sculptor may express him or herself through stone, clay, or porcelain. For the martial artist, his medium is himself, his physical movements and his character traits.

Artistic expression for other artists comes from the expression of their fears, hopes, joys and other emotions. Other artists have the freedom to express the full gamut of mental, physical or spiritual states. A martial artist seeks to develop his physical, mental and spiritual qualities to ever-higher levels so that he or she may express these highly developed characteristics.

Martial arts are indeed a unique art form. They are unlimited by the potential for development of the individual. It is in this endless, shapeless void of self-improvement, enlightenment and quest for inner-harmony that the martial artist finds his medium of expression. Consider this often.

## *Humility*

You cannot develop respect truly without first developing humility. In many ways, humility is the first lesson in marital arts as a precursor to developing respect. There is always someone better than you are. Accept this. Even if you are the best, someone else has useful knowledge that you do not have. If you were able to acquire this knowledge, then you would be even better than you are . . . even if you are already the best.

Humility is another skill that all martial artists must practice. It is the spirit of the martial arts. To have humility means that you have accepted your position and recognized that you are always in a position to improve or gain more knowledge or skill. Until you have this humility, you cannot respect someone better or more knowledgeable than yourself. Without respecting them and opening your mind to what they have to offer, you will not be a true martial artist.

## *Appreciation*

The Koreans call it "Kamsah". When I was a White Belt, I learned the White Belt pattern under the Jhoon Rhee system of American Tae Kwon Do. He named the pattern "Kamsah Hyung". After graduating to Gold Belt, Grandmaster Rhee came to the graduation ceremony to watch the students and speak about martial arts. He explained the simplicity and the significance of "Kamsah Hyung". He explained that appreciation was something that a student must learn to have for himself and to show toward his or her instructor for taking the time and care to share his knowledge with the student.

Learn to appreciate where you are and what you have accomplished. If you stop for a moment to reflect on your level of skill and progress you will have a good sense of where you are and where you should go. If you cannot appreciate what you have gained, then you have gained nothing. Be thankful.

## *The Secret of the Martial Arts*

There is no single, universal secret to success in martial arts. There is no formula for greatness. The secrets to success lie inside each individual.

A thousand martial artists can have a thousand different kinds of success. You cannot have the success of these thousand however; you can only have the success that is yours. You have achieved it for yourself. Do not be afraid that others will take your success because the success is you and your unique journey. It is what you have made of yourself. Success only has meaning because of you and what you bring to it and how it has changed you.

The balance between the physical skill of your body, the mental strategies in your mind and the spiritual development of your character is the true secret to martial arts that is yours to discover.

# Resources

**Books:**

1. The Way of the Martial Artist: Achieving Success in Martial Arts and in Life! - Kevin Brett
2. The Way of Kata - Lawrence Kane, Kris Wilder
3. Achieving Kicking Excellence Series Vols 1 - 10 - Shawn Kovacich
4. Solo Training: The Martial Artist's Guide to Training Alone - Lawrence Christensen
5. Zen in the Martial Arts - Joe Hyams
6. The Fighter's Body: An Owner's Manual : Your Guide to Diet, Nutrition, Exercise and Excellence in the Martial Arts - Lawrence Christensen, Wim Demeere
7. Tao of Jeet Kune Do - Bruce Lee

# Chapter 5

# Martial Arts History and Styles

*"A well-rounded martial artist should have some appreciation of the roots of the thing he is spending so much effort studying."*

Studying marital arts without having some familiarity with the origins of your own style or the history of martial arts in general is like being a member of your family and knowing nothing of your heritage or family history. A well-rounded martial artist should have some appreciation of the roots of the thing he is spending so much effort studying.

## Understanding Martial Arts Styles

There are literally hundreds of martial arts styles originating in countries like Korea, Japan, China, Burma, the Philippines, Okinawa, Brazil and others. At the core of all of the many styles from each of these countries is an approach toward self-defense. (Remember what I said earlier? Martial Arts are about survival). The differences are typically in the general types of techniques that are emphasized in a given style. The founder or creator of a given style developed his style based on some philosophy of defense. Different styles were developed with different influences from their creators.

Some styles are based on animal or insect movements that gave clues to their creators about different styles of movement and defensive tactics. Other styles are based on a philosophy of attack and defense that is built upon by an assortment of techniques intended to defend against certain types of attacks against various types of weapons. The next section describes how some of these styles have evolved into martial arts organizations and what some of the philosophical differences are between styles.

The important thing to take away from this is that there is no one style that is better than another. It all depends upon the self-defense situation, the skill level of the defender and the choice of techniques used in a defensive situation. Do not be fooled by school owners or masters who get involved in heated debates about who's style is best. They are all art forms. Go to an art gallery and decide which painting is the best. It is all a matter of opinion and perspective. I would simply encourage you to study a little bit about several common styles and learn about their general types of techniques and training methods. Different styles are sometimes better suited to different physical builds of people, but this is not always the case. Hit the internet and learn a little before you commit to a style or school. You'll feel more comfortable about your decision once you do choose a school.

| Common Martial Arts Styles | |
|---|---|
| | **Martial Style:** Karate-do and Shotokan<br>**Country:** Japan<br>**Characteristics:** Hard strikes, kicks, block, grappling similar to Tae Kwon Do |
| 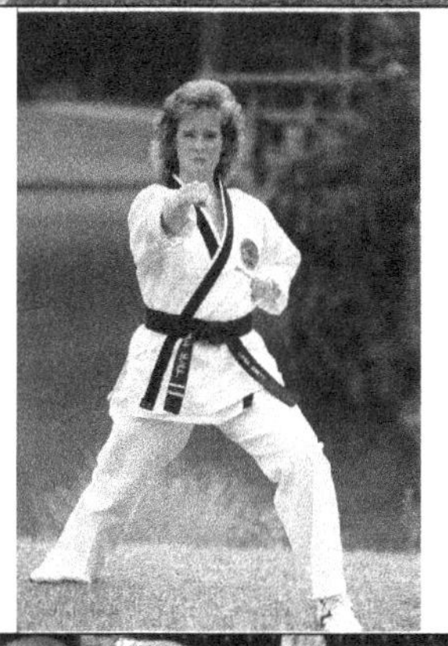 | **Martial Style:** Tae Kwon Do<br>**Country:** Korea<br>**Characteristics:** Punches, many different types of kicks, hand strikes and blocks, grappling, practical schools teach destructive combat application or bunkai of the movements in hyungs (forms or poomse) |
| 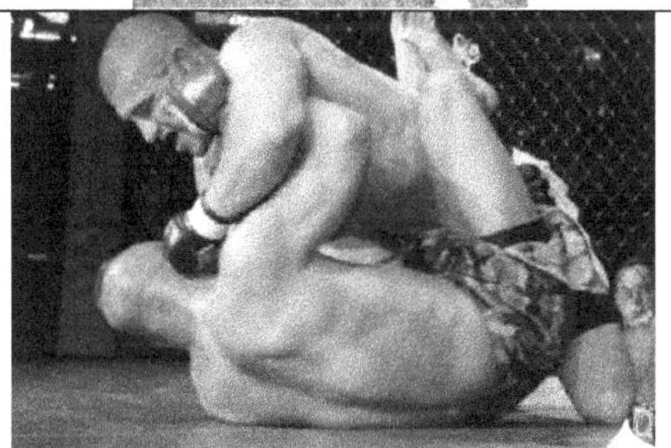 | **Martial Style:** Mixed Martial Arts<br>**Country:** USA<br>**Characteristics:** Grappling, sweeps, throws, punches, kicks, ground fighting |
| 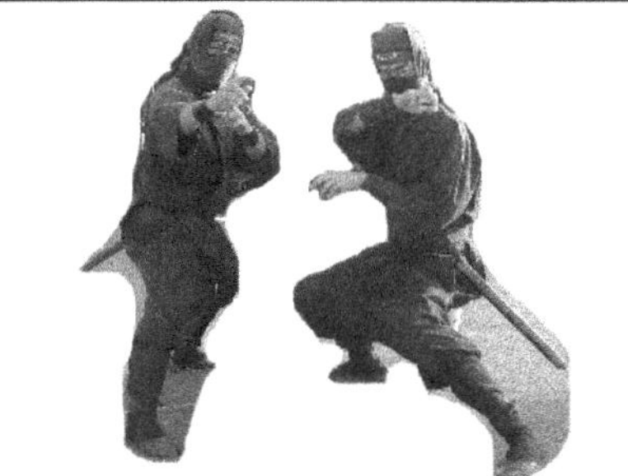 | **Martial Style:** Ninjutsu (Ninja style)<br>**Country:** Japan<br>**Characteristics:** Typically involves basic strikes, punches hand techniques, throws, take-downs, special weapons and tactics |

| | |
|---|---|
| 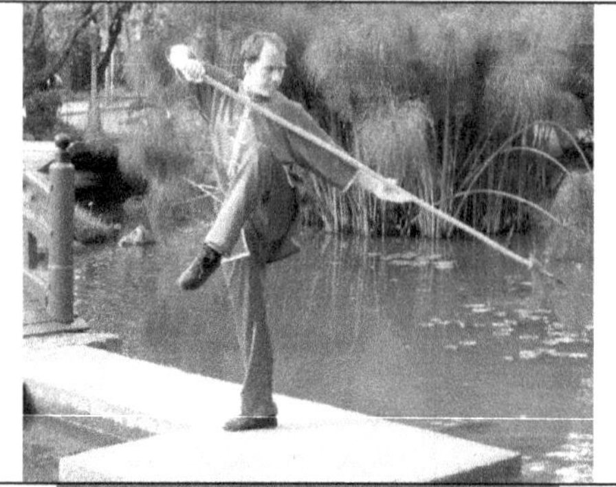 | **Martial Style:** Wushu<br>**Country:** China<br>**Characteristics:** Many weapons and rapid circular blocks and strike combinations mixed with straight blocks and strikes |
| 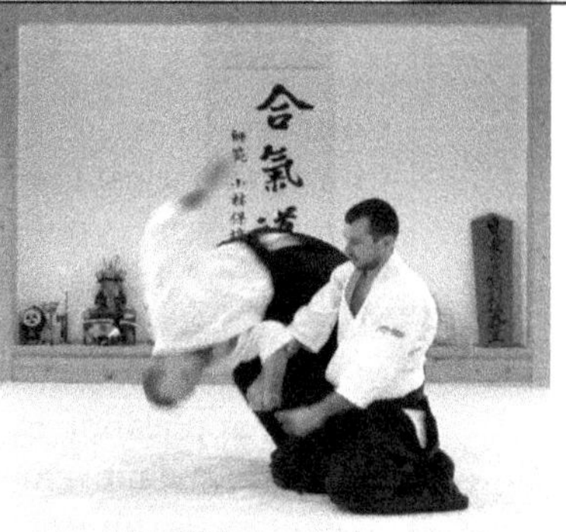 | **Martial Style:** Aikido<br>**Country:** Japan<br>**Characteristics:** Typically non-destructive techniques involving grappling, sweeps and other take-downs and throws, joint locks and joint manipulation, often using your opponent's force against them. |
| 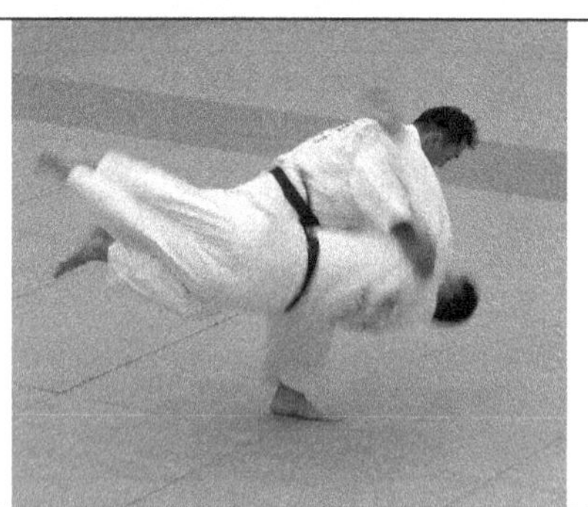 | **Martial Style:** Judo<br>**Country:** Japan<br>**Characteristics:** Grappling, throws, sweeps and other takedowns, ground fighting, joint locks, typically non-destructive techniques |

| | |
|---|---|
| 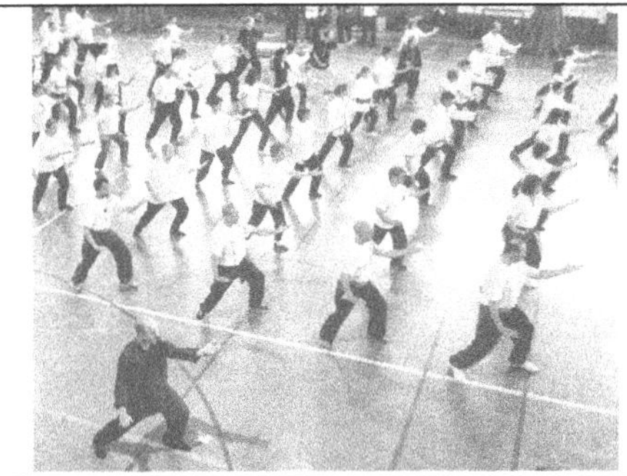 | **Martial Style:** Tai Chi Chuan<br>**Country:** China<br>**Characteristics:** Smooth flowing techniques typically practiced in slow motion, but with combat application. Some styles use the Tai Chi sword and other weapons. |
| 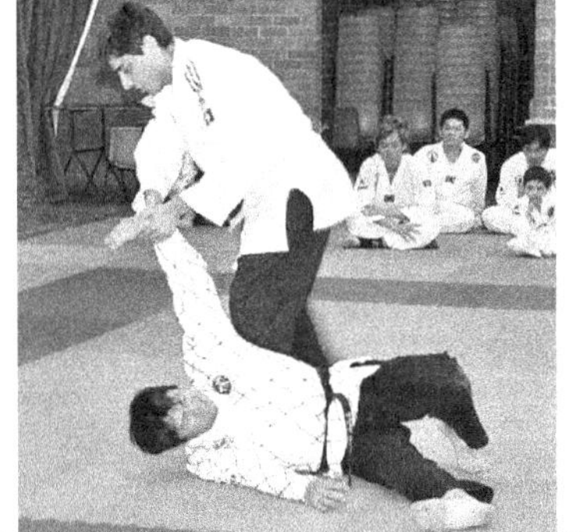 | **Martial Style:** Hapkido<br>**Country:** Korea<br>**Characteristics:** Grappling, throws, sweeps and other take-downs sword, kicks, joint locks and manipulation |
| 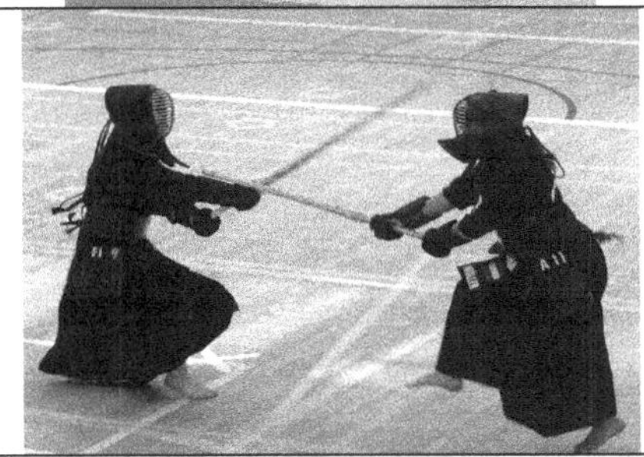 | **Martial Style:** Kendo<br>**Country:** Japan<br>**Characteristics:** Uses the shinai, bamboo practice sword, effectively sport swordsmanship based on Samurai tradition |

## *Origins*

Since the first time that primitive man discovered that he could trip an adversary by sticking out his foot, fighting techniques have evolved, matured and grown into martial arts systems. Throughout its several thousand-year history, knowledge of the martial arts has primarily been transmitted in the oral tradition. At many times in history, martial arts were outlawed in the orient. Consequently, it was not until the twentieth century that many texts on martial arts began to emerge. Since martial arts were illegal to practice during various times in history and in various countries, committing this knowledge to paper was a risky proposition.

Learning technique only does not help a martial artist mature as an artist; it only helps technique mature, not the soul or character. Bruce Lee and Ed Parker have written many outstanding books on innovative technique, training and strategy in the martial arts. Twenty-four hundred years ago the Chinese military strategist Sun Tzu wrote, The Art of War, which dealt with general, strategic concepts of conducting warfare. Sun Tzu's strategies are still in use today and are required reading in most military academies and many corporations. Musashi Miyamoto, considered to be the greatest Japanese swordsman ever, wrote The Book of Five Rings. His landmark work expounded upon the concepts of strategy in swordsmanship in classical Japan. In his day, this was self-defense.

These volumes on strategy share a common theme. They remove many of the specifics and particulars of actual fighting techniques and step back to give the student a broader perspective. They reflect upon the psychology of warfare and combat and the application of the mind, not merely the might. Many of the principles and concepts are valid and applicable in contexts other than martial arts, open warfare or personal self-defense. These seminal works and many others capture some of the core concepts of martial arts and combat. They are part of the ancient and modern history of the art.

It is difficult to say exactly where martial arts began. Ancient Greeks and Romans practiced various forms of wrestling and grappling. We all know of the Roman gladiators and their skill in the arena. The Zulu warriors, the Spartans, the Samurai, the Hwa Rang, the Shaolin Monks and many other warrior cultures are all part of the vast array of cultures and styles that have contributed to the rich heritage of martial arts.

Many sophisticated martial arts techniques and systems were developed in India several thousand years ago. Kaliripayat is one in particular that is still in practice today. As trade routes and the silk roads opened up from China to India, it was only natural that martial arts techniques and knowledge would find its way along these same routes. Martial systems and fighting styles had been evolving in China for several millennia as well. Monks at the legendary Shaolin temple developed a system known as Shaolin temple boxing. Today, Buddhist monks from one of the oldest Shaolin temples travel the world and give public exhibitions of their martial skills.

Legend has it that an Indian monk named Bodhidharma (more commonly Da Mo) left India and arrived some time later at the Shaolin temple in China. There is debate among historians as to whether there was only a single Shaolin temple or several scattered across China. Nonetheless, he arrived at one of the temples and began to impart his knowledge to the very receptive monks.

Da Mo taught fighting techniques to the Shaolin monks. He taught them deep breathing techniques and many concepts related to what we know today as Yoga. He also emphasized the importance of training the mind in meditation. Legend also states that at one point, he spent nine years meditating in a cave sitting facing the wall of the cave watching ants and listening to them scream. As a demonstration of respect, one Shaolin monk cut off his hand and gave it to Da Mo.

The introduction of Indian fighting techniques was a catalyst that spawned a golden age in Chinese martial arts. Innovation and experimentation in Chinese systems helped to continue to evolve the various styles and systems.

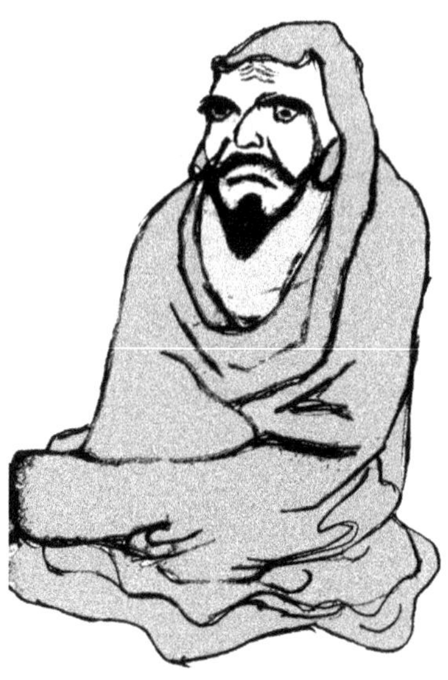

*Bodhidharma*

Monks began to study nature and its effects on the environment for inspiration. They sought a model from which they might derive useful concepts upon which to base martial techniques and systems. Chinese monks studied the effects of wind, rain, fire and water on earth. These were the essential elements and they became known as the five elements. Techniques were categorized according to the elements to which they corresponded. Techniques could be labeled water techniques if they were soft and supple or if they were hard and crashing. An example of water techniques can be found in the Korean Tae Kwon Do variant of Chung Do Kwan meaning Blue Wave School.

Monks also looked to animals and insects. They studied their fighting techniques and survival behaviors to extract useful knowledge. Many Chinese systems arose around techniques that were based on animal movement. Examples that are still taught today include, Tiger Claw Kung Fu, Drunken Monkey Kung Fu, Crane and Eagle Claw Kung Fu.

In China, around 300 B.C, Lao Tzu an ascetic and sage was the first to write down the philosophy of Taoism; the way. Taoism is an ancient Chinese philosophy based upon three core concepts: humility, compassion and moderation. Taoists practice wu wei, the principle of non-action, naturalness. They strive to achieve simplicity or emptiness. Taoists recognize and believe that there is a strong relationship that people have to nature, which leads to greater understanding and enlightenment.

Tzu was a recluse who spent most of his life in nature. Many soft martial arts of China including T'ai Chi are based on his teachings and observations of nature. He recorded these teachings and analysis in his timeless work the ***Tao Te Ching***; the book of changes.

*The weakest things in the world can overmatch the strongest things in the world.*

*Nothing in the world can be compared to water for its weak and yielding nature; yet in attacking the hard and the strong nothing proves better than it, for there is no alternative to it.*

*The weak can overcome the strong and the yielding can overcome the hard; this all the world knows but does not practice.*

- *Lao Tzu*

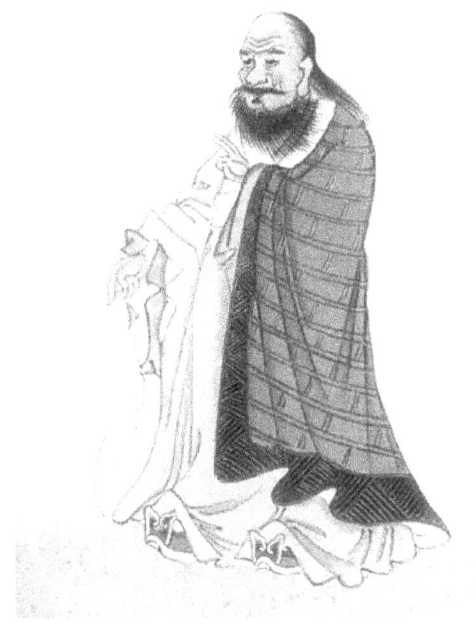

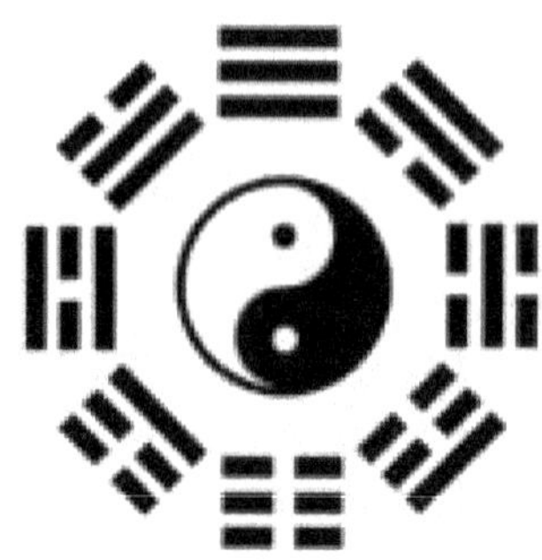

*The Eight Tri-grams of the Pa-Kua*

Names and symbolism of the Pa-Kua

| Name | Attribute | Image |
|---|---|---|
| Creative | Strong | Heaven |
| Gentle | Penetrating | Wind, Wood |
| Arousing | Inciting, Movement | Thunder |
| Abysmal | Dangerous | Water |
| Still | Resting | Mountain |
| Receptive | Devoted, Yielding | Earth |
| Clinging | Light-giving | Fire |
| Joyous | Joyful | Lake |

The table above shows the names, meanings and symbolism of the tri-grams. Pa-Kua means eight diagrams. Many martial arts styles, techniques and philosophies were based on interpretation and application of these concepts and the Pa-Kua served as a unifying symbol of philosophy, enlightenment and martial styles and concepts. The name refers to the eight trigrams that form the foundation of the I-Ching. The I-Ching is a compilation of philosophical works dating back to 800 BC. Parts of it were originally thought to have been written by Confucius, but many scholars today doubt he actually wrote any of it.

The Pa Kua, or Eight Diagrams are an arrangement of symbols composed of straight lines arranged in a circle as shown in the diagram above. These symbols are said to have evolved from the markings on the shell of a tortoise by the legendary Chinese Emperor Fu Hsi, 2852 B.C.

## The Yin Yang

The trigrams comprising the Pa-Kua are said to have been created from the two primary forms represented by a continuous straight line (-) called Yang I, or the symbol of the male principle, and a broken line (- -) called Yin I, or the symbol of the female principle. Mathematics are said to have been derived from the Eight Diagrams, which represent the evolution of nature and its cyclic changes.

The Yin Yang is an ancient symbol. Its oldest existing occurrence is preserved on a metal urn nearly 3000 years old. The outer circle represents the cosmos that contains the Yang (light) and the Yin (dark). The curved line dividing the two signifies the eternal motion of the combined elements, and the small dots mean that even within Yang there is Yin, and vice versa. The whole symbol is the t'ai-chi.

## Martial Arts Philosophy

Confucianism is a related philosophy that asserts that through the training of the mind and embracing the principles of human virtue that you can become a "superior person". Confucianism strives for balance. A central belief is to do the right thing and to have the strength to stand up to people such as tyrants who stand in the way of a better society. A central practice of Confucianism is that you spend time reading and educating yourself, learn the arts, and study individuals who exhibit characteristics that make them true and honorable role models.

Chinese systems often are somewhat of a family affair in nature, meaning that they were often developed by the patriarch of a family and practiced by that family and its descendents. In due time, the Chinese systems, including a vastly rich collection of weapon systems and techniques found its way to the East and South to countries like Japan, Okinawa, Korea, Viet Nam, Cambodia, Burma, Thailand and the Philippines where Chinese based systems blended further with the native systems and fighting arts of those lands.

During much of ancient martial arts history, the martial arts themselves were outlawed at various times. Local warlords who would use trained martial artists in the form of monks from the local temples would then forbid the monks to teach or train others for fear that they would then rise up against the warlord themselves. Because these monks were so highly skilled and their abilities were feared by rival political or military leaders, the penalties and punishments for teaching martial arts were severe and often included execution. It is for this reason that many martial arts system and techniques were often not written down and if they were that knowledge was carefully guarded.

Most martial knowledge was therefore passed on in the oral tradition from instructor or master to student. Often martial arts techniques and systems were disguised to look like exercise, dance or cultural rituals so that they could be practiced without arousing suspicion. Spies would often attend training sessions where martial arts were rumored to be practiced. All except the most senior and trusted students would be taught only symbolic meanings for various movements and not the actual practical self defense application for fear that a spy might be lurking amongst the general population of a training hall where the dance or exercise was being taught. Even in times when it was legal to teach martial arts systems, the true meanings of techniques were usually not taught except to senior instructors because the masters feared their prized knowledge and secret techniques would become common knowledge and thus possible to defeat, hence the shrouded and seemingly mystical nature of martial arts.

## *Fighting Systems and Martial Arts*

Martial arts have a spiritual and ethical foundation and a governing philosophy, fighting systems do not. For example, Krav Maga (a Hebrew term meaning close combat) is the Israeli system of self-defense used by the Israeli military. It is very effective and deadly like many martial arts, but it is a fighting system rather than a martial art. It consists of tactical concepts and techniques, some overall guiding principles for engaging in combat and nothing more. It is highly effective, but it has no philosophical component or spiritual aspect to it.

A martial art may contain philosophical elements that train an artist to avoid confrontation or mitigate risk. It will prepare you to consider carefully the fact that you are about to cause serious or even fatal consequences to an aggressor who is still another human being. By contrast, a fighting system will simply address the fact that an aggressive act has occurred which requires an appropriate physical response. There is no consideration other than to cause maximum damage to the other individual. More of the key elements of character, spirit and philosophy will be covered later.

Every martial art has a ranking system as do some self-defense systems or fighting systems. Many of the Japanese systems are similar to each other. Some of the Korean systems such as Tae Kwon Do are similar to Japanese. The Chinese systems have their own different means of rank and identification.

Every martial artist should at least have some familiarity with other systems.

## *Bushido: Ethics for Warriors*

A Buddhist monk developed a code of behavior and conduct for the Japanese Samurai warriors. The Samurai were the warrior class in feudal Japan. Their code of conduct was known as Bushido - warrior way. The Bushido was essentially a book of manners that described in detail exactly how a Samurai should act in every situation from daily life to combat and in death. Bushido added a spiritual and philosophical component to the fighting techniques and tactics of the various Japanese martial arts that these warriors studied. It was the next level of evolution and maturity toward true martial arts for the Japanese.

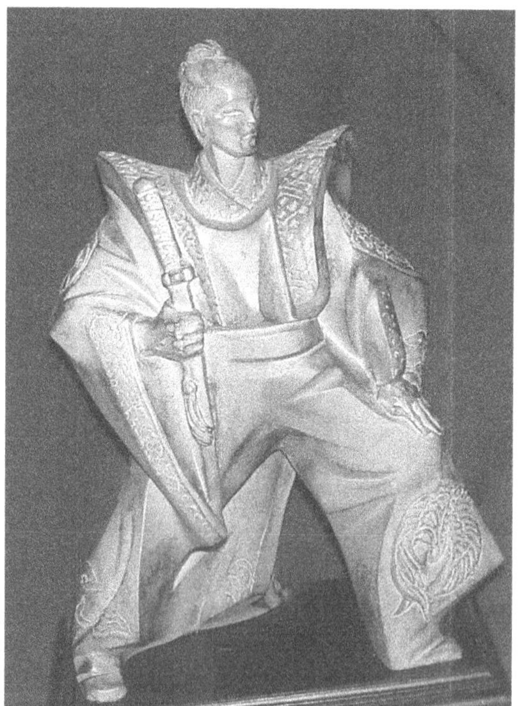

*Samurai in Kabuki theater costume*

Certainly, a system of ethics and etiquette like this was not what the creators of Krav Maga had in mind when they were developing techniques and tactics for neutralizing an aggressor. Bushido was a way of life and it dictated Samurai behavior completely. In Krav Maga the assumption is, there are no rules in a fight. They are two opposite ends of the philosophical spectrum.

Samurai became the educated elite class of Japanese society. They were the ruling class. The fact that Samurai were educated or considered the elite or dominant and controlling class in Japan does not suggest that all Samurai were wealthy. Many Samurai were not wealthy and in fact lived in poverty. However, Samurai were, nonetheless, the only members of Japanese society allowed to wear and use the Samurai swords, Katana, Wakazushi and Daito. You could not train to become a Samurai, you must have been born into a Samurai family; the son of a Samurai. And of course in the patriarchal Japanese society, only men could be Samurai. The Samurai class actually had as many as two-hundred and fifty levels or layers. Those fortunate few who were born into the upper level strata of the Samurai class would fare better in life than those born into the lower classes of Samurai. However, even the lowliest Samurai was higher in society than the highest merchant, artisan or peasant farmer.

## *Warriors and Tea*

There is an old Samurai saying that a man who does not have tea in him cannot truly appreciate beauty and truth. Japanese society evolved highly ritualized actions and activities as part of Samurai life. Every movement was carefully choreographed with painstaking attention to detail and consistency. This highly structured approach to even simple activities was intentionally developed to help symbolize the perfect order and harmony possible in such highly structured situations. These rituals and ceremonies also teach and maintain discipline, respect and order.

The preparation and drinking of tea became the tea ceremony. The finer points of the tea ceremony were taught to Samurai so that they might become more refined in their social graces. The ability to concentrate, and have such a simple pleasure and sensory experience be the focus of so much attention, detail and ritual actually was a training method for Samurai to hone their perceptual skills and ultimately their combat skills. What appeared on the surface to be charm school for Samurai was actually mental training for combat.

The tea ceremony was symbolism for what Samurai strived to achieve in Zen meditation and the practice of their martial skills; eat when you are eating, drink when you are drinking, sleep when you are sleeping. The tea ceremony was codified and refined and practiced in its most minute details with the same attention to detail and refinement that martial artists use when practicing their techniques. The Japanese approach toward many things of importance and reverence was to codify the rules, processes and behaviors of key aspects of daily life.

*A fourteenth century Samurai*

These ceremonies helped to underscore the importance of the event in the lives of Samurai and other citizens. The order brought about by ritualizing and formalizing activities like tea ceremonies emphasized the importance and desirability of order in the universe and in life. Order is good. Structure is good. Disorder and lack of structure is bad.

The shape and form of the Samurai class evolved from the ninth century until its culmination in the nineteenth century. In its last few centuries, the Samurai became the military and governmental elite in Japan. As part of that class, it became required and expected that Samurai were well-educated, possessed social graces, were capable of artistic expression and of course were skilled in martial arts.

Samurai were taught and practiced flower arranging, they learned musical instruments and music composition, they pursued studies in painting, calligraphy and poetry. Why would warriors need to know these things? How do these practices relate to combat and martial arts?

Like many modern military academies, the Japanese wanted and expected their Samurai to be well educated and well rounded in their skill, knowledge and abilities. For Samurai to truly be the elite, they must be on a par with those considered to be the elite in most other societies especially those in the West. The pursuit and practice of these various art forms and activities also helped the Samurai practice focus, concentration and attention to detail. Samurai learned patience and perseverance through a variety of outlets.

By contrast, modern martial systems are not focused on culture and artistic endeavors such as flower arranging and the tea ceremony. A recent addition to the martial world, for example is the United States Marine Corps Martial Arts Program (MCMAP). This innovative system with its slogan of "One Mind, Any Weapon" has a wide variety of specific close-quarters combat techniques. MCMAP is indeed a true martial art with both a philosophical and moral/ethical element to it as well as physical conditioning and specific martial techniques and weapons – no flower arranging.

MCMAP also has a system of various belt ranks, and stresses mental and character development, teamwork, leadership, citizenship and the responsible use of force. All Marines are required by the Commandant of the Marine Corps to earn their Tan belt; the first rank. Any Marines deployed in theaters of combat are required to earn their gray belt; the second rank, and all infantry Marines are required to earn their green belt. The program is designed to help the Marines to develop the mind, body and character simultaneously and equally.

The Marines study martial history and culture. They have required reading including the Art of War and master a variety of rough terrain skills. Studies examine societies that produce warriors either primarily or exclusively. Examples include the Apache Indians, the Spartans and the Zulus.

These ancient martial styles continue to find new life and new application in modern life and help modern warriors prepare for and fight the conflicts of the twenty-first century by building on the techniques and concepts of several millennia of martial heritage.

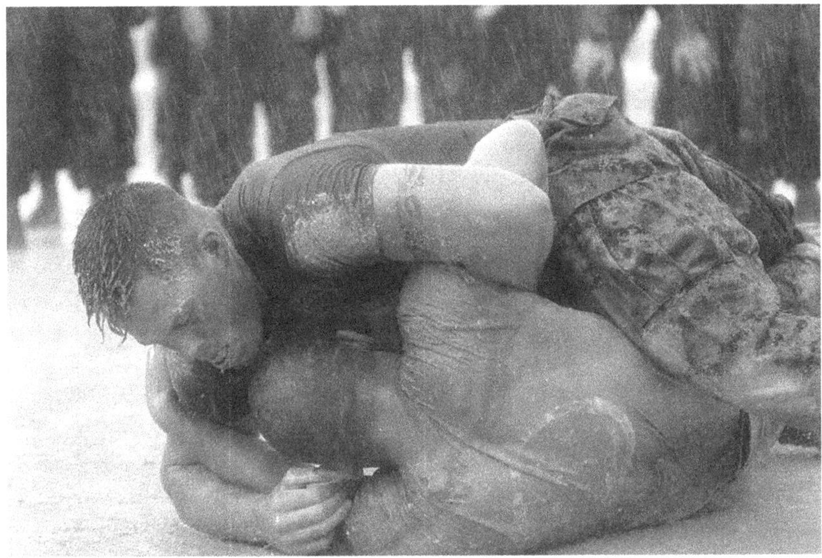

*U.S. Marines practicing ground fighting in the rain as part of the MCMAP.*

## *Musashi Miyamoto*

A martial education would not be complete without some familiarity with this truly legendary figure. Essentially he and Sun Tzu's Art of War were the inspiration for this book. One of the most famous Samurai was Musashi Miyamoto. Musashi wrote ***The Book of Five Rings***, which described the approach and strategy of studying the sword and combat strategy in general. His book has applicability on many levels and in many disciplines. Today almost every business school and office supply store has copies of this book in the business section. It is timeless and like a truly good book on strategy, always just beyond the complete grasp of the student. His concepts, their application and interpretation are always subject to more discussion, analysis, re-interpretation, and evaluation.

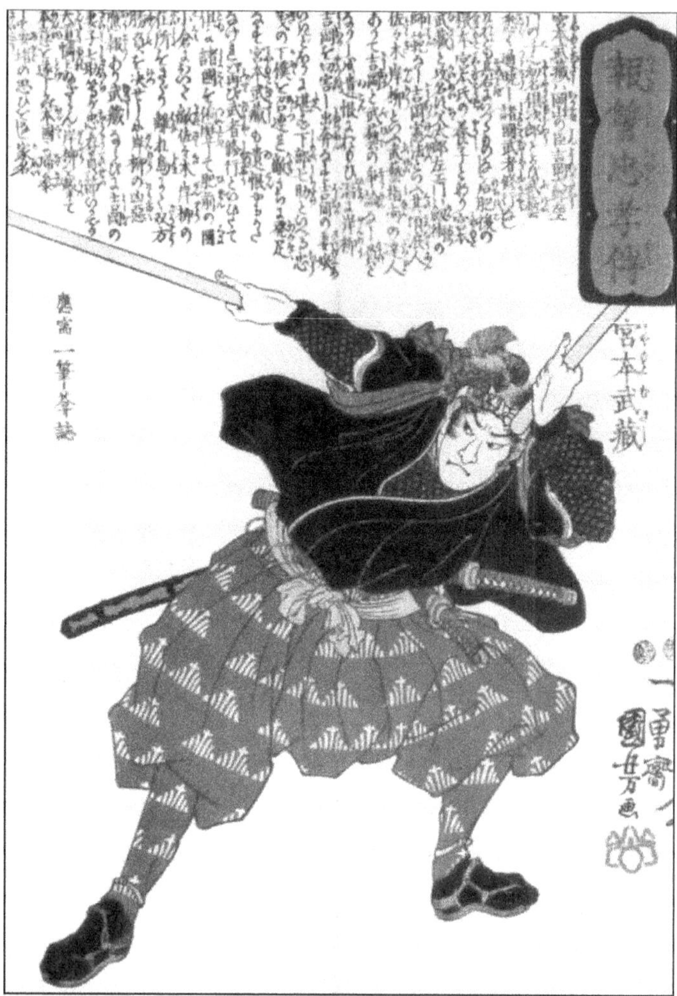


*Musashi Miyamoto*

There are many stories and legends surrounding Musashi. He favored the bokken, the wooden training sword, over an actual metal blade. Legend states that he defeated at least sixty opponents in mortal combat to prove the superiority of his style of swordsmanship. His most famous legend is the story where a prince in a wealthy Samurai family challenged him. The prince was highly skilled in swordsmanship. The two agreed to meet at a specific time on a nearby island where they would dual to discover the superior swordsman. The prince was punctual. Musashi overslept, and on the boat ride to the island as he allegedly recovered from a hangover. He fashioned a primitive bokken from an oar using a knife. He arrived several hours late to find the prince furious. The two faced off and with one blow, Musashi's bokken felled the prince. Musashi returned to the mainland. He spent the last several years of his life writing his Book of Five Rings.

## Hwa Rang Warriors

While the Japanese shaped and evolved their elite Samurai warrior class, Korea developed an elite band of highly skilled, highly educated warriors called the Hwa Rang. One of the under belt patterns in the traditional Chon Ji Hyungs (patterns) developed by General Choi, the founder of the International Tae Kwon Do Federation is named for these famous warriors.

The Hwa Rang studied history, the arts and sciences. They were expert in martial arts and were skilled in wilderness survival techniques. They trained for brutal conditions and in extreme types of weather. The Hwa Rang were the "Warriors of Flowering Manhood." They swore loyalty to king and country. Hwa Rang were the Korean equivalent of the Japanese Samurai. Both Hwa Rang and Samurai were Asian counterparts to the European knights who also strived for high levels of conduct, morality and virtue to compliment their warrior training. These are many of the same qualities shared by the ancient Spartans and their warrior culture.

Throughout history and across nearly all continents there have arisen cultures of warriors who have sought to enhance and enlighten their existence and their pursuit of lethal combat skills. In fact the pairing of social graces, artistic expression and moral underpinnings with the most primitive of human behaviors - that of mortal engagement with another being seems almost an intentional, if not conscious effort to tame, balance and counteract these primal almost animalistic behaviors with something seemingly more human certainly on a higher plane of existence.

## *T'ai Chi Chuan*

Many of us have seen people practicing T'ai Chi. We think of it as moving meditation, a graceful exercise for older citizens. Few know that it is a martial art and that each movement has a practical and lethal application in self-defense just as do the kata of the hard-styles. The Chi refers to Chi energy and the ability to control and direct this energy and maintain it. T'ai Chi makes use of the centers of the body; the upper center, the middle center and the lower center. These are the centers of balance, of power, and spirit.

It is useful for you to practice their kata in slow motion as a T'ai Chi practitioner. This way you may discover the subtle movements and aspects of your techniques and improve and focus on their details. T'ai Chi, when applied at normal speed in self-defense is as effective as any style of martial arts in providing self-defense. It is even rumored that Genghis Kahn studied T'ai Chi and understood its combat application.

Unfortunately, many who study T'ai Chi today are not even aware of its rich martial heritage and simply focus on its symbolism and meditative aspects. This is much the way other martial arts are taught in the more commercial settings. The true meaning and combat applications are lost. Regardless of the style or system of martial arts you may be studying, the following chapters provide fundamental concepts, skills, strategies and character development that will help you become a more successful martial artist and person.

## Ninjas

Japanese Ninjas are certainly the stuff of legend and the subject of many movies, but the reality is that they were skilled in a wide variety of unconventional weapons and tactics. Ninjas existed for hundreds of years in Japan and were the original Special Forces commandos. Ninjas were masters of disguise, camouflage, concealment, explosives and deception. Ninjas learned and trained in a variety of close combat techniques drawn from various more established Japanese arts. They served as intelligence agents and assassins. With these skills and capabilities, Ninjas have left an indelible mark on history and earned a key place in the history of martial arts. In fact, it could be argued that Ninjas have played a significant role in martial arts history and because of their diversity of techniques and tactics and effectiveness, they have served as the blueprint for all modern Special Forces and many intelligence agencies and their operatives. Navy S.E.A.L.s, in particular, employ a wide variety of special weapons, tactics, explosives, concealment, stealth and other skills directly attributable to Ninja operations.

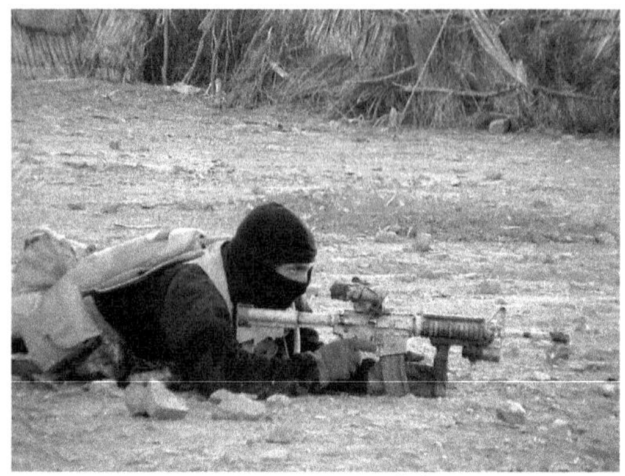

U.S. Navy SEAL in Afghanistan

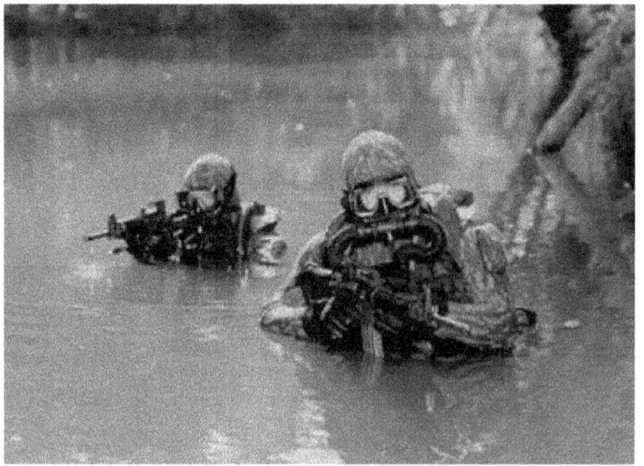

SEAL underwater gear

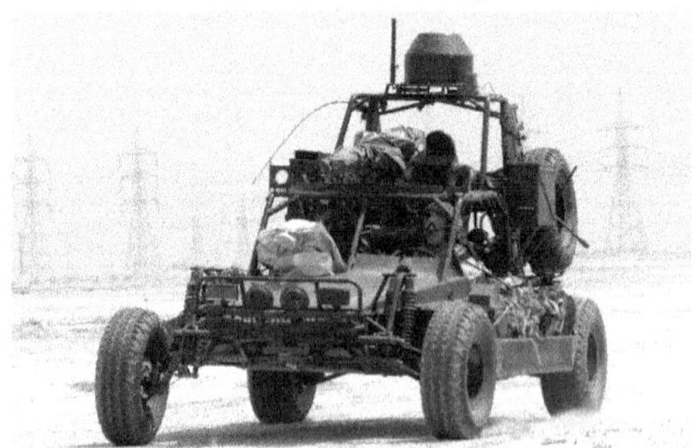

SEAL
Desert Patrol Vehicle

*Not your typical Ninja equipment!*

## The Legend of the Belts

In ancient times martial arts students began their studies with a white uniform and a white belt. The belt was used not only as a symbol of rank, but to hold up their pants as well. Many martial arts classes were held outdoors or in a Dojang that may have had only a dirt floor. As students continued in their studies, their white belts would begin to turn yellow with the sweat from their workouts. As they worked outdoors in the grass, rolling, flipping and practicing take downs, their belts would take on green stains. As the students worked during the course of several years their 'white' belts became more soiled with blood, dirt and mud. Eventually, when the student tested before the headmaster of the school they would be presented with a black belt if they passed. At that point students were allowed to also wear black uniforms if they choose.

As students progressed from beginning levels to expert level, their belts became darker. After reaching the black belt level a student was then beginning all over again on a higher level. Black belts would train, study and teach to reach higher levels of knowledge, proficiency and martial skill. As the new black belt began to wear with age, it would fray and show the white material inside of the belt reminding even the most experienced black belts that they are all still white belt students inside.

Today we use a colored belt system to signify the level of skill of progress of the student. The belt colors get progressively darker as the student works towards the black belt level. The black stripes on the belt are used to mark a student's progress in their requirements for their belt level.

Earning a new belt in the martial arts is a significant achievement for anyone. Students should always remember that unlike many other things in life, a new belt in Karate is not automatic or guaranteed; it must be earned, the old fashioned way, with hard work and determination: Nothing really worth doing is ever easy, but the rewards are certainly worth the effort required.

Always treat your belt and other student's belts with respect. Tradition has it that a student should never wash their belt because that would be like washing out the sweat and work that went into earning it! Of course you should always wash and press your uniform as a sign of respect to your instructors. Your uniform should be treated with respect because it is a training tool and a part of your martial arts equipment. All of your martial arts equipment, manuals, videos, bags, uniforms, sparring gear and weapons should be kept in neat clean condition. Keeping your equipment in ready condition helps students develop the necessary discipline required to always be prepared.

## Typical Meanings for the Different Belt Colors

In most martial arts systems that incorporate colored belt ranks, there are various meaning associated with the particular colors of the different belts. The table below includes common meanings of the belts in the Tae Kwon Do family of styles. There are many variations, but this should give you some idea of the concept of progression of knowledge, skill and maturity.

| | |
|---|---|
| **White** | The student is pure or without knowledge of Tae Kwon Do. |
| **Yellow** | Symbolizes the student, likened to a seed, is beginning to see the sunlight. |
| **Orange** | Represents the full power of the sun, or knowledge which will help the seed take root. |
| **Light Green** | Represents the seed beginning to grow. |
| **Dark Green** | Shows the young seedling flourishing. |
| **Blue** | Designates the young plant reaching for the sky. |
| **Purple** | Represents the clouds of rain which feed the plant and give it life. |
| **Red** | Signifies Danger. The student has good technical knowledge, but still lacks control and discipline. |

| | |
|---|---|
| **Brown** | Symbolizes closeness to earth, or a better understanding of one's mind and body. |
| **Black** | Means no fear of the dark, or an understanding of the art. There are 9 degrees of Black Belt. When all the above colors are combined in equal amounts, they come out black. Black represents the combination of all of the knowledge gained from all of the belts which come before. |

Since Take Kwon Do is the most widespread style in the United States and for the most part, around the world, I have provided a brief history of this art.

## *History of Tae Kwon Do*

More than 2000 years ago in southern Korea a new martial style emerged which would eventually become the most prolific martial art in the world. Tae Kwon Do was originally known as Taekyon. It is a native Korean form of punching, kicking, and parrying with an opponent that encompasses many open handed style combat techniques. Today Tae Kwon Do is studied and practiced by more people than any other style of martial art.

Tae Kwon Do is not merely a fighting style. It is a system of training the mind as well as the body. The strong emphasis on moral and spiritual development of the character of the martial artist is consistent with all martial arts. Humility, respect and self-discipline are key character traits that all martial artists seek to develop and maintain.

Regular practice of Tae Kwon Do provides students with excellent workout benefits. When performed with good technique and power, Tae Kwon Do techniques can be devastating to the attacker. Tae Kwon Do is considered to be one of the easiest martial arts to become proficient in, but like all other martial arts can take a lifetime to master. Tae Kwon Do's power comes from its simplicity, making it one of the most practical martial arts.

Tae Kwon Do is a combination of the hyung (pattern or form) style of practicing technique from its predecessor styles of Taekyon and Subak (also known as Soo Bahk Do), and the kata (formal exercises) of the Okinawan Shuri-te and the Naha-te schools of karate. Tae Kwon Do is famous for its beautiful but deadly aerial kicks. It is considered a hard style martial art even though many of its movements are very fluid and graceful. Tae Kwon Do includes the sharp straight-line movements of karate and the flowing, circular movements of kung-fu and tai chi.

Early settlers arrived in what is now Korea after the Neolithic Age; (roughly 10,500 - 300 BC). These ancestors of the Koreans, like many other primitive cultures, played different games for entertainment and practiced various religious rites.

Some of these early games were Yongko in the Puyo state, Tongmaeng in Koguryo (northern Korea), Muchon in Ye and Mahan and Kabi in the south dynasty. These were games that were practiced as part of religious rites. Over the centuries, training exercises were developed based upon these games. These exercises served the dual purpose of improving one's health and endowing the practitioner with martial arts skill. The fighting art of Taekyon, the forerunner of modern Tae Kwon Do, evolved from these exercises.

2000 years ago the Korean peninsula was divided into three separate kingdoms. These were the Silla Kingdom and the Paekche Kingdom in the south, and the Koguryo Kingdom in the north. Archeological evidence indicates that Tae Kwon Do dates back thousands of years. For example, during the Koguryo dynasty a painting on the ceiling of the royal tomb of Muyong-chong depicts two men wrestling. They are clearly in a recognizable Tae Kwon Do stance. The Koguryo dynasty lasted from 3 AD to 427 AD. It is reasonable to conclude that Koreans began practicing Tae Kwon Do at about this time.

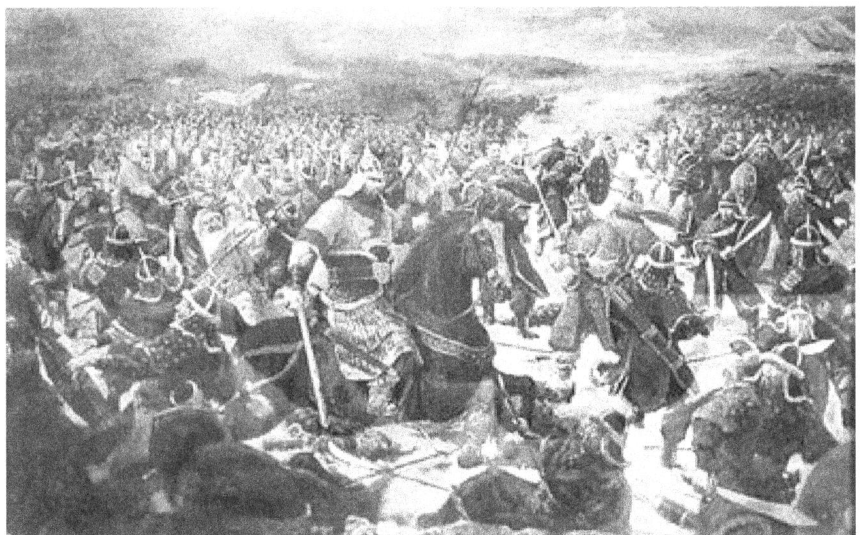

*The battle of Salsu (612 A.D.) between the between the Kingdom of Koguryo and the Sui Kingom a the Salsu River in Korea*

South of Koguryo in the Silla Kingdom, Tae Kwon Do was widely practiced from about 668 - 935 AD. The Silla Kingdom was established about 50 years before the Koguryo Kingdom. Again, we see evidence of Tae Kwon Do being practiced at Kyongiu, the ancient capital of Silla. There, figures of two giants facing each other in a Tae Kwon Do stance appear on the Keumkang Ginat Tower at Sokkuram in Pulkuk-Sa Temple.

In 688 AD the Silla Kingdom won a decisive victory in a long struggle among the three kingdoms. After the country was unified under a single government, from 688 until about 935 AD, a Golden Age of prosperity and enlightenment followed. It was during this Golden Silla Age that a group of warriors emerged who would change the face of martial arts history. Korea's rough equivalent to the Japanese Samurai warriors, this fierce group of warriors in Silla were known as the Hwarang warriors. Hwarang-do (the way of flowering manhood), included training of mind and body. These warriors dedicated their lives to studying classical writings, hunting and martial arts.

In 935 AD the kingdom of Silla was overthrown by a Korean warrior named Kyonghum. Kyonghum created the kingdom of Koryo. It was from Koryo that the Western name Korea was derived.(Note: The Koryo form happens to be a traditional Tae Kwon Do requirement for WTF 1st Degree Black Belt) From 935 to 1392 AD Tae Kwon Do continued to be the dominant martial art in what is now Korea during the Koryo dynasty. During this time,

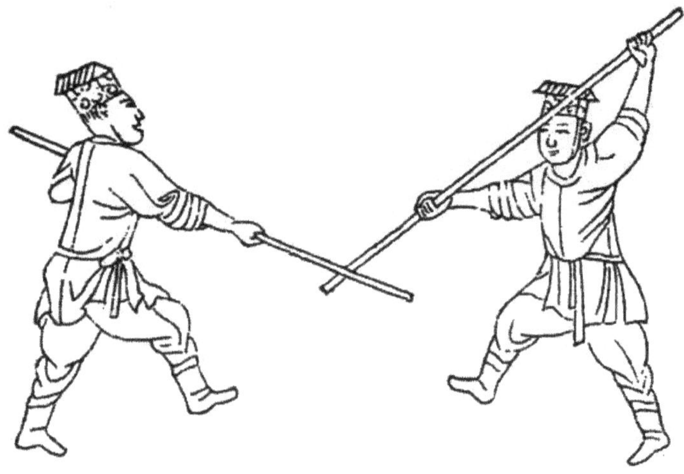

*Korean warriors ca. 1786 practicing with the staff*

Subak, another native Korean martial art, enjoyed the height of its popularity as both a sport and martial art. At the same time in neighboring China, during the Sung and Ming dynasties, Kung Fu's popularity spread.

The history is vague, but, it is possible that interactions between the peoples of Okinawa and Korea resulted in the Okinawans learning Subak. This would then make Subak the Okinawan predecessor of Okinawa-te which then evolved into the Okinawan style of Kara-Te (literally Chinese hand, and later just meaning open hand).

Subak was chiefly practiced by the military during the Korean Yi dynasty (1392 to 1907) and was in fact an entrance requirement for the military. Tae Kwon Do received a royal boost when King Chongjo published a textbook, Maye Dobo Tongji, on martial arts with a chapter on Tae Kwon Do. Diminishing royal support for Subak as the official martial art of the military caused widespread practice of the art to drop off. Subak became merely a sporting pastime.

During the Yi Dynasty the Hwarang warriors were disbanded and training in Hwarang-do was forbidden. Learning and higher education were the order of the day and military arts practice was not a priority of the Yi Dynasty.

Still, many of the Hwarang warriors continued their training in secret in Buddhist monasteries and in remote parts of the country. In this way Hwarang-do was kept alive. During the Japanese occupation of Korea (1909 - 1945), martial arts practice in Korea was outlawed. Martial arts practice in Korea was done in secret and passed on from father to son in the context of the forms or hyungs.

After World War II and the end of the Japanese occupation of Korea, Hwarang-do reemerged and has been established world wide. During periods when martial arts were discouraged or outlawed in Korea, many practitioners left for China and Japan where martial arts practice was allowed. There the masters of Taekyon were exposed to Chinese styles such as Kung Fu and Japanese styles.

A synthesis of these new techniques with existing Taekyon practice resulted in a fragmentation of styles of Taekyon. Because the different masters of Taekyon went their various ways, they each had their different encounters with other styles. These encounters had the effect of causing the masters to modify and augment their styles.

After World War II the divergent Taekyon masters returned to Korea. There they joined the national movement to revive Korean traditions, culture and martial arts. Many of these masters started their own schools.

The kwans or schools of Tae Kwon Do were born at this time as the masters of these new styles established their schools. Jhoon Rhee was the first to accurately document (1969 Action Karate) the development of the Kwans in Korea. Master Rhee is the father of American Tae Kwon Do.

According to Jhoon Rhee the first five Kwans were: Chung Do Kwan(1945), Moo Duk Kwan, which taught Tang Soo Do (1945), Yun Moo Kwan (1945), Chang Moo Kwan (1946), Chi Do Kwan (1946). Several more Kwans were founded after 1953 and in the early 1960s. The chart below show the major Kwans of Tae Kwon Do:

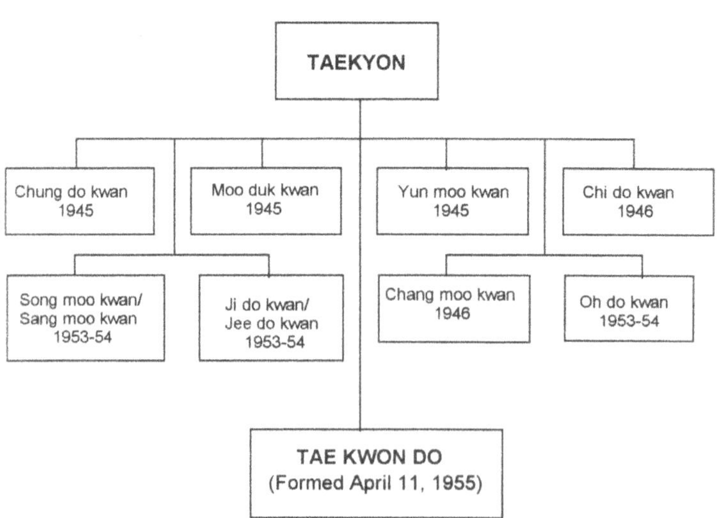


*The eight original Kwans of Tae Kwon Do*

In 1945 the new Korean military was established. Choi Hong Hi, then a second lieutenant in the army, began teaching Taekyon to Korean army troops. Later Choi gave Taekyon demonstrations during training in Kansas which was the first exhibition of this style in the United States.

A movement developed from 1945 to 1955 to unite the martial arts of Korea into one system. Finally, in 1955, a conference of Chung Do Kwan masters adopted the term Tae Kwon Do coined by Choi Hong Hi, who had risen to the rank of general. The name was chosen by General Choi because of its similarity to Taekyon.

In 1952 a demonstration was given to Korean President Syngman Rhee. As a result of this demonstration Syngman Rhee decreed that all Korean soldiers be trained in the martial arts. In 1954 General Choi Hong Hi developed a center for Taekyon training for the Korean military on the island of Che Ju.

In 1961, by order of the new military government, the Korean Tae Kwon Do association (KTA) was established with General Choi Hong Hi as its first President. The KTA established national standards for black belt certification.

General Choi sent Tae Kwon Do practitioners to many countries to internationalize the art. Jhoon Rhee was the first to introduce Tae Kwon Do in the United States in 1956 at San Marcos Southwest Texas State College. He was attending college where he taught a non-accredited Tae Kwon Do course. In 1958 he founded his first public Tae Kwon Do club in San Marcos.

Tae Kwon Do proliferated in Korea from the military to the public school system. Many public Dojangs were established and Tae Kwon Do was accepted as a required part of physical education training in the public schools.

General Choi Hong Hi founded the International Tae Kwon Do Federation in 1966, resigned from the KTA and moved to Saskatchuan, Canada.

The South Vietnamese government asked for help from General Hi to provide instructors to teach their troops Tae Kwon Do to help in their struggle with the North Vietnamese. Tae Kwon Do spread to other parts of the Pacific rim, Europe, the Netherlands and the Middle East.

In 1968 Tae Kwon Do made its way to Britain, Spain, Belgium, India, Yugoslavia and Hungary. In 1973 the World Tae Kwon Do Federation (WTF) was established back in Tae Kwon Do's home country of Korea. In 1974 the U.S. Tae Kwon Do Federation was formed.

Jhoon Rhee invented the original safety chops for competition sparring and eventually opened the first Tae Kwon Do school in the former Soviet Union after the fall of Communism. He was also a major influence in the movement to make Tae Kwon Do an Olympic sport.

Under the direction of General Hi, Tae Kwon Do has spread to more than 62 countries. It is estimated there are 15 million Tae Kwon Do practitioners, far exceeding any other single art. In 1975 more than 700,000 were reported to be practicing in the U.S alone. Today there are many millions Tae Kwon Do students in the United States!

In 1980 the International Olympic Committee (IOC) recognized Tae Kwon Do as a legitimate Olympic sport. As a result Tae Kwon Do was a part of the Olympic Games in Seoul Korea in 1988 with the United States Olympic Tae Kwon Do Team taking the gold medal!

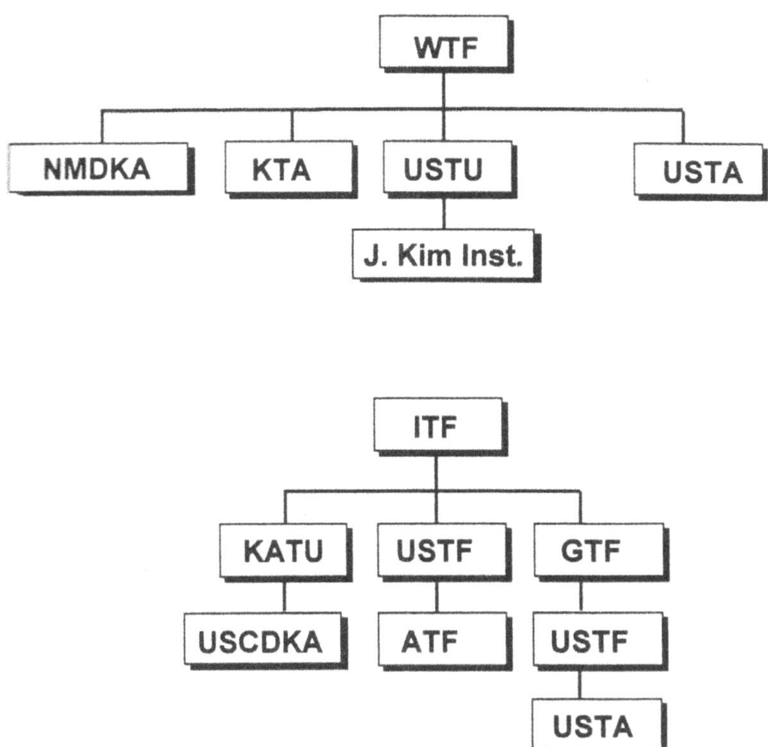


*Tae Kwon Do Organizations*

**Internationally Recognized:**

- ITF - International TKD Federation (Chonji forms)
- KATU - KoreAmerican TKD Union (Chonji forms)
- GTF - Global TDK Federation (Chonji forms)
- USTF - United States TKD Federation (Chonji forms)
- USTU - United States TKD Union (Tae Guek & Pal Gue forms)
- WTF - World TKD Federation (Tae Guek & Pal Gue forms)
- KTA - Korea TKD Association (Tae Guek & Pal Gue fo.Luts)

**Nationally Recognized:**

- USTF - United States TKD Federation (Chonji forms)
- USTA - United States TKD Alliance (Chonji forms)
- ATF - American TKD Federation (Chonji forms)
- USTA - United States TKD Association (Tae Geuk & Pal Gue forms)
- ATA - American TKD Association (Sang Anm forms)

## *The Korean Flag and Its Symbolism*

There is a meaning and a history associated with the Korean flag. The flag of South Korea, designed after World War II and the end of the Japanese occupation of Korea.

During the Japanese occupation of Korea, martial arts practice was forbidden and Korean culture and art were eventually outlawed by the Japanese. After the defeat of the Japanese in 1945 the Korean government took many deliberate steps to revitalize Korean arts, culture and nationalism.

The Yin Yang is the center of the Korean flag. The Chinese Yin Yang is often black-and-white and aligned on a vertical axis with one small black dot in the middle of the white element and a small white dot in the middle of the black element. The Korean Yin Yang is aligned on the horizontal axis. Instead of representing the opposites of black and white or dark and light, the Korean Yin Yang represents the opposites of Water (blue) and Fire (red).

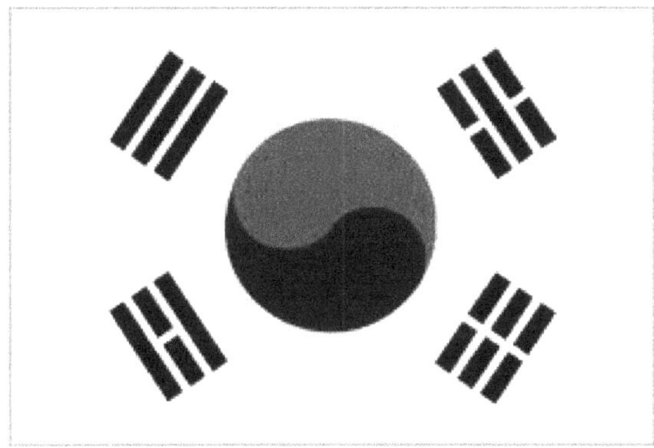

*Korean Flag*

The four trigrams circling the Yin Yang have their roots in Chinese Philosophy taken from the I-Ching or "Book of Changes". The meanings of the four trigrams are as follows:

Top Left - Heaven
Bottom Left - Fire
Top Right - Water
Bottom Right - Earth

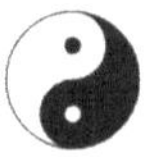

# Resources

**Books:**

1. The Way of the Martial Artist: Achieving Success in Martial Arts and in Life! – Kevin Brett
2. The Original Martial Arts Encyclopedia: Tradition, History, Pioneers – John Corcoran, Emil Farkas
3. Martial Arts of the World: An Encyclopedia (2 Volume Set) – Thomas Green (editor)
4. The Spirit of Aikido – Kisshomaru Ueshiba
5. The Ninja and Their Secret Fighting Art – Stephen K. Hayes (the first actual American Ninja)
6. Ninjutsu: History and Tradition – Dr. Masaaki Hatasumi (34th Grandmaster of the Togakure Ryu – Ninja School)

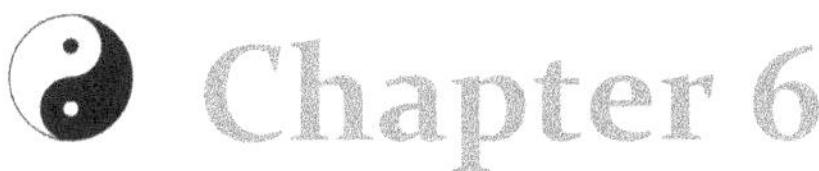

# Shopping for a Martial Arts School and Style

*"Rank means nothing if the knowledge of these 'Masters' cannot help you achieve your goals."*

## Reasons Adults Study Martial Arts

At this point in the book, I've taken you through a journey covering the history of the martial arts, given you some insights into what it means to be successful in martial arts and how that can transcend every aspect of your life. I have provided a foundation for beginners in understanding the key elements of training of your body, mind, character and spirit. I have also provided an overview of the differences between some of the major styles to give you a better idea of your potential options depending upon where you live. There's only one thing missing - a place to do all of this and an instructor to take you on your journey to black belt and beyond.

So you're looking for a martial arts school or maybe you're looking for a school for your children. Either way there is a reason or motivation behind your desire to find a school. Understanding what you are looking for will make it easier to know when you have found it. As you begin your quest to find a suitable martial arts school that will meet your needs and expectations you will have many questions. There are many useful checklists in this chapter of what questions to ask instructors and yourself before you begin your personal journey into the martial arts.

The difficulty in shopping for a martial arts school is that as a non-martial artist, you are not qualified to evaluate the quality of the instruction. Assuming that your have no knowledge of martial arts, the information in this book will give you what you need to find a good school and to develop a better appreciation for what the martial arts are about.

What many potential students of martial arts focus on first are location, price and amenities. Yes, you want a school that is reasonably close to work or home and certainly you do not want to have to break the bank to afford it, but these are not the most important features. The quality of the instruction is paramount. You will be spending three or four days per week there if you are serious about improving and gaining what there is to gain, so ask a lot of questions; visit a lot of schools many times before making a choice. At the same time, keep in mind that sometimes your first martial arts school is like your first boyfriend or girlfriend. They may seem nice at first, but there's also a chance they just might not work and you should not let that negative experience keep you from trying again.

Shopping for a martial arts school is exciting and a little scary too. It's important to keep in mind that there are a wide variety of schools. A champion can be born in any environment. A school is simply a place to study and in the more traditional sense, it can even be outside where you don't even having four walls around you. Your school may be a garage or a corner of a gym or wherever. Don't think that the only schools worth attending are those that have the appearance of a modern club-like setting. While their appearance and accommodations may be tantalizing, the quality of instruction may not be of a high caliber.

There are literally hundreds of martial arts styles from many countries. Pick up any copy of the Yellow Pages in any medium to large metropolitan area and you will likely see dozens of advertisements for martial arts schools. There are masters, grand masters, champions, world champions, senseis and sifus. There is Kung Fu, T'ai Chi, Judo, Tae Kwon Do, Shotokan, Aikido, Brazilian Jiu Jitsu, Karate Do, Kendo, Hapkido and many other "Do's" How can one sort them all out and begin to understand how to proceed?

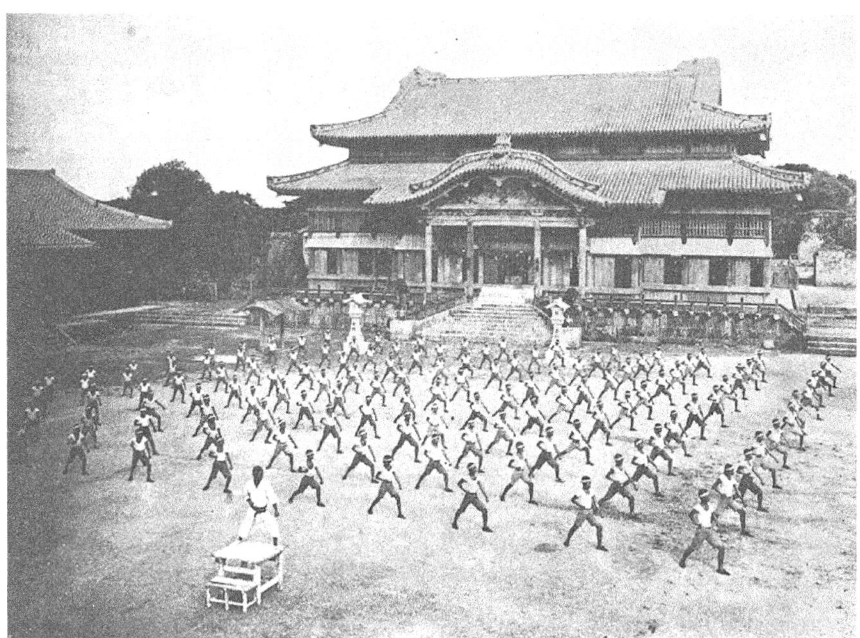

*A Traditional Martial Arts Class at Shuri Castle in Japan 1938 – no walls or cappuccino bars in this dojo!*

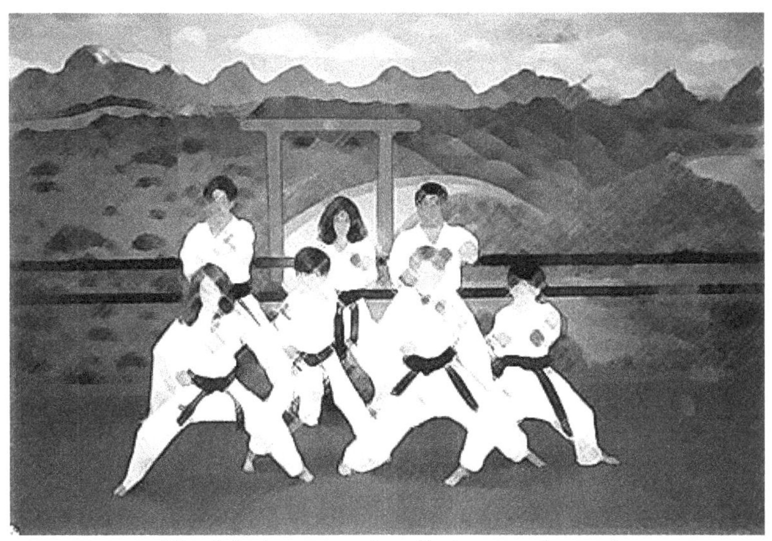

*Black belts come in all sizes and ages!*

Let's begin with understanding why you are looking for a martial arts school. What got you interested? What do you expect to get out of martial arts? There a number of reasons that people typically seek martial arts training for themselves or their children. In the box below are a few common reasons.

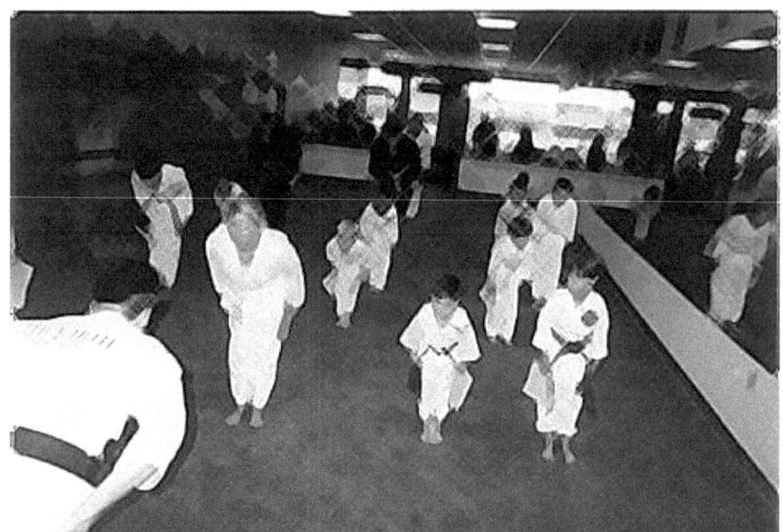

*Respect and confidence are key qualities*

## Reasons Adults Study Martial Arts

1. I want to learn to defend myself.
2. I want a total body workout that includes cardio kickboxing instead of the typical workout at a local gym or health club.
3. I want to develop self-confidence, self-esteem, self-discipline.
4. I want to study martial arts traditions and styles as an art form.
5. I'm interested in Mixed Martial Arts (MMA).
6. I want to compete in martial arts tournaments.
7. I want to lose weight and get in shape.
8. I want to learn to become more focused (hey even adults need focus and structure!).
9. I want to become better at setting goals and achieving them.
10. I want to learn more about traditional martial arts values and ethics: humility, respect, honor, determination, perseverance, etc.

You may be motivated by one or more of these reasons or even something completely different. Regardless, there is a multitude of benefits to be gained from the study of martial arts. Take a few minutes and review the list above and identify which reasons are your main motivators. If your motivation is not on the list, write it down. Think these through and ask yourself, why the selected items are motivating you. I just want you to be sure of why you think you're interested in studying martial arts before you begin your search for an appropriate school.

## Reasons Children Study Martial Arts

For our children, the common reasons for studying martial arts are similar. Parents may have motivations similar to those above and probably a number more as in the box below.

### Reasons Children Study Martial Arts

1. I want my child to learn to defend himself/herself.
2. I want my child to become involved in a vigorous physical activity.
3. I want my child to develop self-confidence, self-esteem, self-discipline, respect.
4. I want my child to learn more about goal setting and personal achievement.
5. I want my child to learn traditional martial arts values and ethics: humility, respect, honor, determination, perseverance, and strength of character to stand up to peer-pressure or to confront bullying.
6. I want my child to learn to become better focused to help him or her out in school and to develop valuable life-skills.
7. My child needs more structure! (Don't we all!)

Again, review the list above and make sure you have a complete understanding of the reasons why you want your child studying martial arts and also what they're interest is. Often children will be motivated by television shows and movies they have seen where characters display impressive martial arts skills. If those are the visions they have swirling in their heads as they begin a martial arts program, so be it, as long as you, the parent, realize that the martial artists performing the stunts in the movies didn't learn those techniques overnight.

These two lists of reasons are pretty much carbon copies of virtually every advertisement you will ever see for any martial arts school. Somewhere in the promotional materials for any self-respecting school will be these key values, benefits and selling points. You the shopper must beware because while almost every school will claim to meet these needs, not all will really deliver the goods. Don't just assume that it's an automatic; insist.

This chapter will help you better understand what you should look for and ultimately what your study of the martial arts should include. If you study martial arts as they have been studied for centuries and learn the many qualities and skills that a true martial artist seeks to develop, you will achieve all of the objectives identified in the previous lists and have a rich and rewarding future in the martial arts.

At this point you have a list of reasons why you are interested in martial arts and what you hope to get out of it. Something to keep in mind, however, is that martial arts and martial arts schools are not silver bullets. By that I mean that the instructors and curriculum and are not miracle cures for all that ails you or all that you hope to achieve. They can provide encouragement, structure and educate you to varying degrees on the basic values and qualities that will help you satisfy your needs. You will need to do much work to develop any skill, level or knowledge or personal qualities to reach the goals you have set for yourself or your child. Do not put all the burden or responsibility on the shoulders of your martial arts instructor. Before you start looking for a martial arts school there are a few more things you will need to consider in the following sections.

## Martial Arts Benefits

In this section we'll take a brief look at benefits of martial arts study. I've already touched on many of the common benefits and outcomes that many people hope to gain from martial arts for themselves or their children. When you begin calling around or visiting martial arts schools I strongly recommend you make a list of your specific reasons. What is your "Why?" Whether you are shopping for yourself or your children, first make certain you know just what you are looking for. Review the list below and add any other reasons, benefits or desired outcomes you hope to gain from your adventure into the martial arts.

**General Benefits of Martial Arts**

1. Self-Confidence
2. Self-Defense
3. Self-Discipline
4. Physical Fitness
5. Improved focus and concentration
6. Respect for authority and others
7. Self-Respect
8. Achievement and Goal Accomplishment
9. Improved preparation and planning habits

The benefits listed above are just the highlights. If you recall the virtues discussed in chapter 2, there are many direct and indirect benefits to martial arts study for both children and adults.

Now you have given it some thought and hopefully have a better idea of what you are seeking. Let me assure you that once you find a suitable school, regardless of what reasons you have for studying the martial arts, I am certain you will find it invigorating and rewarding on many levels and you may even realize some benefits that you had never anticipated.

One side benefit of my study of martial arts is that when I first enrolled and earned my white belt, there was a very attractive blond in my white belt class who had signed up at the same time. She apparently had her eye on me while I was only focused on martial arts and developing the strength and stamina to continue on through the ranks with as much ease as she seemed to move along. Four years later we were married and four years after that we opened the United Karate Institute of Self Defense, Inc. in Alexandria, Virginia with three other instructors - not a bad side benefit. Certainly, I had not ever expected that signing up for martial arts would lead me to owning and managing a school and meeting my future wife. Signing up for martial arts was the best decision I ever made!

## *Qualities of a Martial Artist*

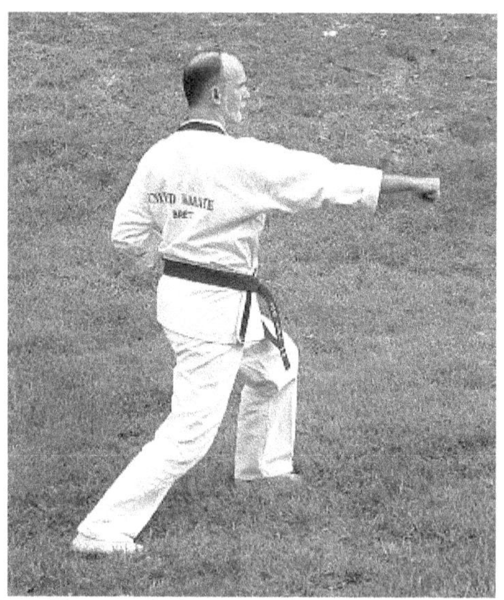

*A well-rounded martial artist must learn about and focus on the following general topics of study:*

**Martial Arts Topics for Study and Development**

- Martial Arts Origins and Traditions – *appreciation for the past*
- Skill and Training – *training the body*
- Strategy and Tactics – *training the mind*
- Spirit and Excellence – *training the soul and character*
- Success for Life – *foundations for the future!*

Within each of these general topic areas are dozens of sub-topics that make up the body of knowledge that a martial artist must learn and practice. It is a journey of a life-time and it can be life-changing. Martial arts really are about becoming what you were meant to be. Through martial arts training and the development of essential qualities, the potential for human development and achievement is unlimited!

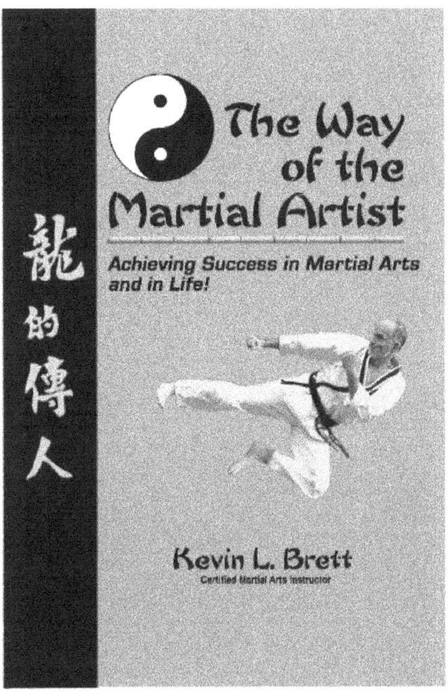


Coincidentally the topics above are the chapters of my book ***The Way of the Martial Artist: Achieving Success in Martial Arts and in Life!*** I wrote that book because I wish I had a book like this when I began my martial arts studies. I would have progressed faster and farther and that is why I wrote it for my students.

This book describes all of the essential qualities of a martial artist through each of the chapters in the box above and explains what these skills, techniques, strategies and concepts are to help you become a much better educated and enlightened martial artist. Feel free to go to my web site to read the actual Table of Contents, Foreword, Preface and Introduction. http://www.KevinBrettStudios.com

## *Martial Arts Instructors*

As with school teachers, doctors, pilots, and any other profession, all martial arts instructors are not created equal. First of all, you have to remember martial arts are just that - an art form. Martial arts schools are not federally or state controlled. There is no consumer watchdog agency to ensure the quality or legitimacy of martial arts instruction. There are no national standards, criteria or requirements for martial arts. This is both a blessing and a curse. Essentially anyone can open a martial arts school after obtaining a business license. Decent schools have instructors with a reasonable idea about what they are doing with their art and their teaching ability and at the same time also understand how to run the school as a business so they can pay the rent and keep the lights on. That being said, what does that tell you about their martial art, their ability to teach what you are looking for and the actual benefits that you will receive from studying with them; nothing much.

In the previous section there were a number of questions that I asked you answer about yourself and your reasons for wanting to study martial arts. In this section we'll address some of the questions you need to pose to the martial arts school instructors and owners

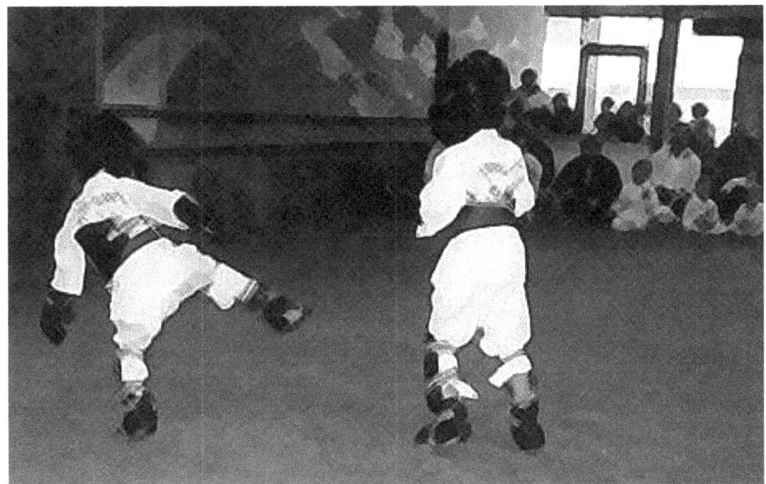

*Mini-warriors learn control and self-discipline under pressure*

First a few rules of thumb to consider: You will encounter many Masters and Grandmasters. Schools and their advertisements will tout their owner's amazing achievements in martial arts competition or in rank achievement. Many school owners will be high-ranking black belts such as 5th degree black belt up through 10th degree black belt. Every martial arts style has a slightly different scale of belts or colored sashes and ranks. Don't let this confuse, impress or intimidate you. Think of it as nothing more than some one who has gone through elementary school, then on to middle school, high school, college and possibly graduate school. ***Rank means nothing if the knowledge of these "Masters" cannot help you achieve your goals.***

All schools will claim to teach the standard fare: discipline, self-confidence, respect, etc. All schools will try to impress you with the qualifications and accomplishments of the owner or master, however, you will almost never be taught by that person, but by his or her junior instructors – often times you may be taught by an 18 year old who is a 1st degree black belt or sometimes even a brown belt. There is nothing inherently wrong with this as long as you do receive some instruction from higher ranking black belts as you increase in rank over time.

Some schools will tout the fact that they belong to some national or international association or federation related to their martial arts style. This is not a bad thing, but it is not a guarantee that you will receive quality instruction or that there will be good focus on self-defense or other key studies.

Most schools will try to fit you into what programs they have to offer. You want to try to pry more info out of them on how they will fit your needs and specifically how they will meet the claims that they make. Finally keep in mind that martial arts schools are not miracle factories. You will have to work and put a lot into it in order to get a lot out of it.

## Questions for Martial Arts School Instructors

1. How many instructors are on your staff?
2. What are their ages and qualifications or ranks?
3. How long have they been with you? (good schools will be good at retaining qualified and motivated instructor staff)
4. Are there any non-black belt level instructors teaching such as brown belts or red-belts? In other words, how much black belt instruction will I actually receive?
5. How do you train or qualify instructors? Are instructors simply those who have earned black belts or have they been through any type of instructor certification or training program beyond their basic black belt rank achievement?

Keep in mind that many schools may be staffed by one or two full-time instructors or school managers while the rest of the teaching staff is composed of part-time black belts who may not have been through any type of comprehensive instructor training or certification. This is where my comment earlier about all instructors not being created equal comes in. You must keep in mind that even if an instructor is certified by some means under someone that simply means they have had some type of training program that they have passed or through which they have earned some type of certificate. It does not mean they are skilled at teaching, gifted, motivated or even very competent. I must stress the importance here of visiting schools and watching several classes and how the different instructors interact with students at various belt ranks and skill levels. If a school will not allow you to observe

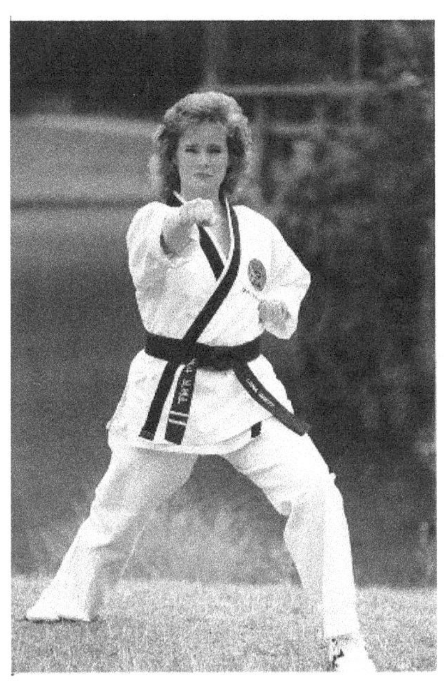

their classes or answer questions about their instructors you probably want to pass on that organization.

Any martial arts instruction should emphasize discipline and respect toward instructors and toward students as well as self-discipline. Instructors should be like an encouraging coach. There are times to be tough and times to be inspiring and motivating; watch for this. It is important to discuss with the instructors how they handle discipline. What methods do they use? Do they consider or handle input from parents, school teachers or other concerned parties. Discipline is important to reinforce respect and to provide boundaries for what is acceptable behavior, but it should not become an open door for verbal abuse or demeaning students. ***Discipline should be a learning experience and have a positive outcome that helps the student grow from the experience.***

While experience is important it is not the only thing that makes a good instructor. At United Karate we had one junior instructor who was eighteen and a first degree black belt. He was gifted with motivating children and keeping them under control, engaged and focused. Adults were also inspired by this young man. We put him through our 13 week instructor training and certification program complete with a 130 question practical exam. He was a better instructor than many higher ranking black belts I have come across.

In the box below is a list of some desirable traits you would hope to find in a good martial arts instructor. You will not necessarily find these qualities in *every* instructor, but during the course of your studies you will likely learn from multiple instructors and more senior martial artists and black belts. Make note of these qualities in the various instructors you encounter to determine which qualities you find most important and how the instructors seem to fit into these categories.

## Instructor Qualities

1. Focused – doesn't get sidetracked from the lesson plan or the point that he or she is making.
2. Motivational – encourages everyone to dig deep and to want to work hard to improve.
3. Technically competent – must know the curriculum and be able to explain and break down techniques, kata/forms and all important strategies and concepts.
4. Knowledgeable – should have a reasonable grasp of the differences between major martial arts styles such as Chinese styles (Kung Fu, T'ai Chi), Korean Styles (Tae Kwon Do, Hapkido, Tang Soo Do, Mu Duk Kwon) Japanese Styles (Karate Do, Aiki Do, Kendo, Jiu Jitsu) Brazilian, Pilipino and so forth.
5. Disciplinary – able to maintain order, keep attention of the students, commands respect.
6. Technically skilled – able to demonstrate any and all techniques and concepts the way they should be performed.
7. Detail oriented – able to focus on small details of technique and performance.
8. Traditional – able to draw upon martial arts history, traditions and values and teach respect, humility, perseverance and many others essential qualities that all martial artists must develop.
9. Instructors may or may not be in excellent physical shape, but they should be able to teach students how to properly execute techniques. Although it is generally a good sign when an instructor leads by example and is able to do exercises with the class at times. At other times it is important that the instructor is walking around observing as the class performs the exercises so that he or she can watch for proper technique and motivate students.
10. Some instructors will expect students to condition themselves outside of class so that class time can be used to teach techniques while other instructors will use class time explicitly to help students physically train and condition. Both approaches have their pros and cons.

11. Good instructors explain the mechanics of movement and the physics of each technique. If they simply tell you to imitate them then you will never understand what you are doing and are likely to injure yourself.
12. Instructors should ideally be able to demonstrate one or more lethal applications for any technique in a kata, unfortunately many were only taught some watered-down explanation for a technique or some symbolic interpretation. EVERY technique in a kata is for combat purposes. The ancient masters did not waste time or motion with fluff or superfluous techniques. To gain a better understanding of the concept of Bunkai (interpretation of kata), read my book or buy a copy of *"**The Way of Kata**"* by my friends Lawrence Kane and Kris Wilder. This book explains the REAL purpose of martial arts kata which 99% of commercial instructors are never taught.
13. Treats students with respect and encourages with positive motivation.
14. Love teaching martial arts and never tire of teaching.
15. Continue to improve their knowledge, skill and ability.

## *Studying Options*

Your martial arts studying options will be determined by the geography of where you live. Some areas will have a wider variety of options than others. Nonetheless, schools and training options can be generally categorized as shown below. Match these training options up to your reasons for studying martial arts from earlier in this chapter to get an idea of what you will be searching for in terms of a training experience.

**Martial Arts Study Options (types of schools)**

1. Traditional Schools
2. Modern Schools with Sport Emphasis including mixed martial arts
3. Blended schools – with attention toward tradition, but also coverage of sport, competition, fitness training and self-defense applications
4. Self-Defense focused
5. Fitness-focused – cardio kickboxing
6. Weapons-focused schools/styles

## *Martial Arts Organizations and Associations*

There are many martial arts clubs, associations and organizations in existence today. Many of these organizations function as the caretakers of their various styles and keep close watch over the teaching of these styles and the standards of performance and advancement.

It is important for students to understand the importance and the role that these organizations play in the martial arts world. To better understand the structure and role of these organizations it is useful to step back for a moment and consider the evolution of martial arts systems.

The martial systems that we study today are largely derived from systems that were developed by individuals. These individuals developed systems of self-defense, gave them names, refined them and began to teach them to others. Students of these instructors were the proving ground for these martial systems and the masters continued to refine, innovate and evolve their systems and styles. As the systems developed into maturity, various ranking schemes evolved with most of them. Students were identified by their rank and instructors could gauge their ability even without personally knowing the student. As more curriculum came into being, higher ranks were possible. Students who stayed with a master for a long enough time could rise in rank and skill as the master's own skill expanded and the curriculum with it.

Various systems adopted sophisticated philosophical and spiritual bases upon which they built their techniques, strategies and customs. Like any family tree, the martial arts family tree has many branches in many countries. Each time a senior instructor would leave a master, he would go to another location, teach what he had learned and in many cases modify, innovate and adapt his original system into a variant of what he had mastered. In some cases, major innovations came into existence by the hard work, analysis and creative insight of masters who devised systems that were significantly different from what they had originally learned.

Morehei Ueshiba, the founder of Aikido (meaning "Harmony Way") built his system based on the philosophy that he respected his opponent and therefore wished no harm to his adversary. The original techniques that he developed caused no permanent harm to the adversary. There were no strikes or kicks that would inflict damage that would prevent an opponent from recovering after a time and coming back to continue an assault. I believe that philosophy, although honorable, is not a practical basis for a robust system of self-defense. Opponents will get up and return to the fight, at least until the defender has shown through enough attempts that he is impervious. Conversely, the general strategy in Kenpo Karate is to cause maximum damage in a complete flurry of devastating techniques. These styles of martial arts are on opposite ends of the force continuum.

Later variations of Aikido began to incorporate some number of simple kicks and strikes for use on a limited basis for persistent attackers. Later students of Ueshiba and his son developed these variations and they are now part of the martial family tree.

Tae Kwon Do and all of the other major and minor systems of martial arts have evolved, branched and morphed into a myriad of flavors all having some common elements. It is part of the martial tradition for a senior student to leave his master, go on his own, reflect and adapt and hopefully devise some useful innovations or potentially even introduce a radically new style or system. This keeps the arts dynamic, vibrant and growing.

In modern times, along with the development of new styles and systems comes the evolution of martial arts organizations and associations. These organizations charge membership and testing fees and provide some degree of quality assurance over their domain. Students derive a sense of legitimacy by receiving black belt certifications from them. Aside from revenue generation for the leaders of the organizations, certification and rank testing are usually promoted as providing acceptance for the students. If you obtain a black belt from organization “A”, then you will be recognized anywhere that organization has a school or club. The problem with the recognition or certification is that many organizations refuse to recognize each other. These organizations typically require students to re-test on material that is very similar.

Often one organization may look upon black belts from another similar organization as being illegitimate. There are politics and egos involved and many organizations have come into being simply because the leadership of one organization had a falling out or fundamental differences so a divergence occurred and several new organizations then came into existence.

Another inconvenient feature of the organizations is that they periodically make subtle changes in the curriculum and the expected way in which the students are to perform the material. This is solely for requiring instructors to attend teaching seminars and to act as a control mechanism so that the organization maintains control over its affiliate schools. There are no practical, martial reasons for example, in changing how many Kihaps (yells) there are in a pattern, or on which moves they are to occur. This keeps instructors and students on their toes with useless and frivolous changes where time could be better spent focusing on the Bunkai (practical combat application), which most organizations do not teach or even know.

What are the advantages of these modern martial arts organizations? There is robust curriculum; however lacking it may be in specific focus on self-defense. These organizations are prevalent, instruction is usually consistent, and instructors do receive thorough training, which improves the student's experience. However, these martial organizations are highly politically charged often with much in-fighting. Self-defense and street survivability is often covered as more of an afterthought or an adjunct to the traditional curriculum, whereas if the focus were on the interpretation of the kata (Bunkai), then students would be learning what the movements of the patterns could do rather than learning to mimic a specific performance for purposes of passing a belt test. I have seen master-level classes where self-defense is not even discussed except in academic terms, not because there is any practical consideration of the need for it. The result, I believe, is students who are highly trained and tested in the tradition, etiquette, symbolic meanings and history of the kata and proper performance of techniques, but uneducated in the adaptation of these techniques and practical application for survival.

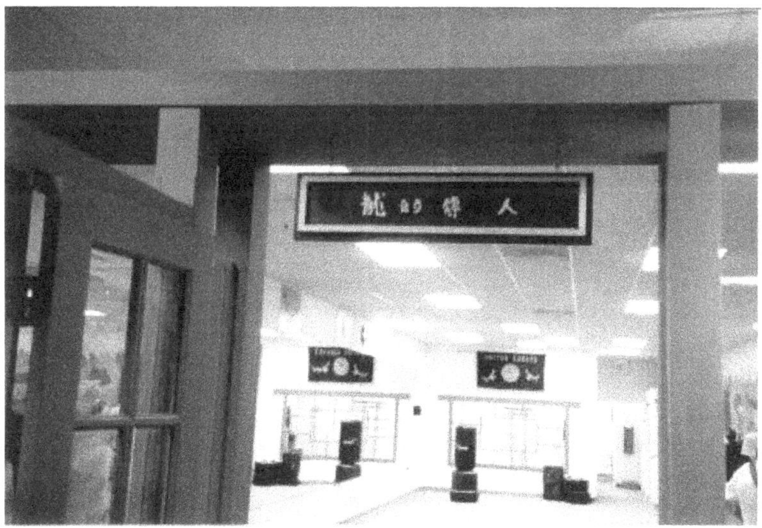

*A view from the front entrance at United Karate. The weapons room is in the rear. The lettering is Chinese for "People of the Dragon" signifying wisdom, maturity and restraint.*

It is important for students to understand the importance and the role that these organizations play in the martial arts world. To understand better the structure and role of these organizations it is useful to step back for a moment and consider the evolution of martial arts systems.

## Martial Arts Schools: Physical Layout

Martial arts schools vary in physical appearance, layout and accommodations greatly, but essentially a martial arts school is a big empty room. In fact, if you recall the photo of the Shuri Castle in Japan at the beginning of this chapter, you don't even necessarily need a room. Your dojo may be outside. Some schools are nicer, cleaner and equipped with more accommodations than others. But always remember that the quality of the instruction is the key factor. Location is probably second because you don't want to have to drive too far or you may be less motivated to stick with it. Some things that you may find or look for in a martial arts school are listed below.

### Martial Arts School Accommodations

1. Bathrooms
2. Showers
3. Padded floors or large floor mats for throws and ground fighting
4. Large mirrors so that you can see how your techniques look
5. Weapons on racks (swords, bo-staffs)
6. Computerized billing and record keeping
7. A school web site
8. Customized school uniforms, gear and sports apparel
9. A pro shop
10. Books or videos for the school's curriculum
11. Weight equipment and other exercise equipment
12. Saunas and tanning beds
13. Handouts of the curriculum for each level
14. School vans for after school pickup (some schools have after school programs where they will help students with their homework
15. Adequate seating in the lobby – you will be spending time waiting for your children. Make sure you have a place to sit.

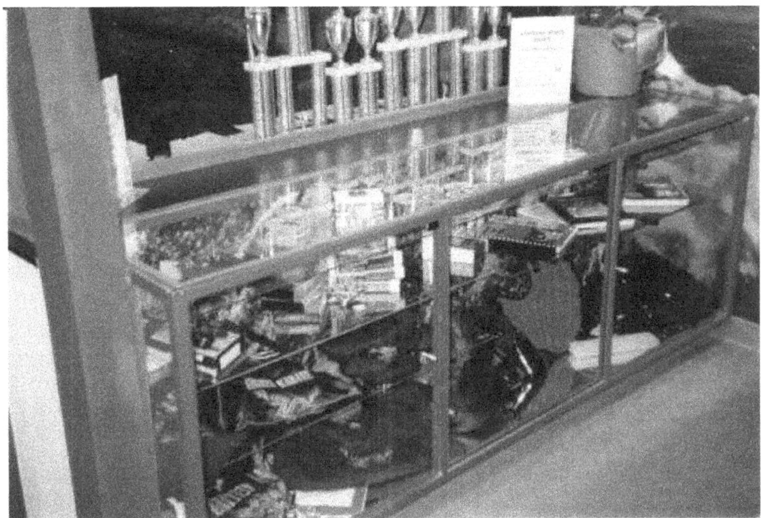

*A display case with United Karate jackets, sparring gear, curriculum videos, student manuals and other goodies!*

The essentials are simply a clean, safe room and the basic kicking and punching pads. It is not necessary to have a sauna, tanning beds or a juice bar or even showers. You will pay for these extras as part of your tuition. This leads to my next point: Where to find martial arts schools.

## Where to Find Martial Arts Schools

1. Shopping malls
2. Strip malls
3. Universities
4. Asian book stores
5. Bulletin boards in martial arts supply stores
6. Churches
7. YMCA/YWCA
8. Community centers
9. Civic centers
10. Classified ads in newspapers
11. Yellow pages
12. Internet searches
13. Roadside signs
14. Word of mouth
15. Oriental restaurants
16. Local Military Bases
17. Local Police/Sheriff Departments

## *Martial Arts Programs*

Before we discuss different types of programs that schools offer, let's talk about how schools might be run. Below are some key aspects of how a school might be structured to operate:

Individual classes for children and adults (occasionally, though, ages might be combined once or twice per week particularly on Saturday's when the schedule is shorter.

Flexible schedule. For example if you are a yellow belt your schedule should offer a variety of times so that you can pick the

| Sample Class Schedule | |
|---|---|
| Monday | 5 PM |
| Tuesday | 6 PM |
| Wednesday | 7 PM |
| Thursday | 8 PM |
| Friday | 5 PM |
| Saturday | 9 AM |

days and times that fit your schedule. For any given belt rank, the schedule will vary something like the example above so that no matter what rank you are, you will have some variability in your schedule.

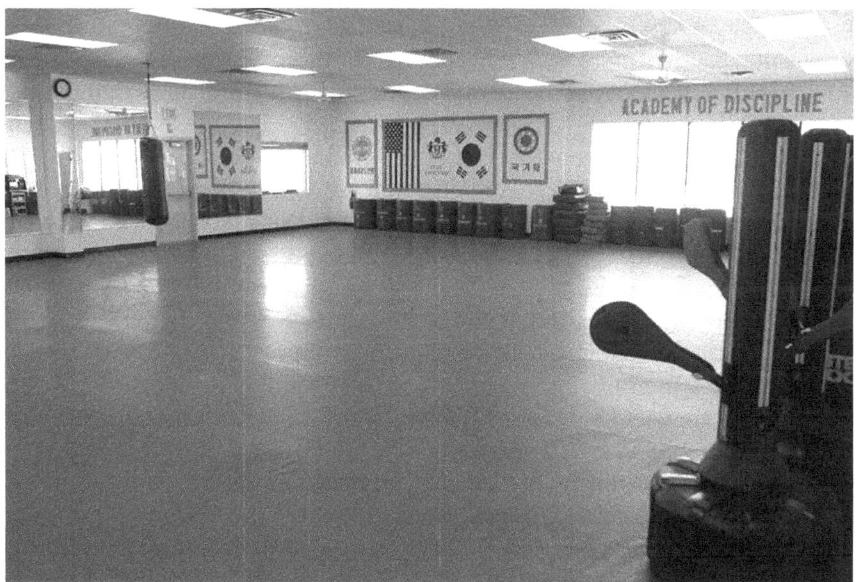


*A typical Tae Kwon Do Dojang; flags, mirrors, pads, kicks pads along the far wall – the basics*

## School Program Features

1. Free intro class: Some schools have some type of introductory offer to allow you to have two or three classes or more so that you can try it out to see how you like the school. Often the intro offer will include a free uniform. However, the free uniforms are generally very light weight and inexpensive, so don't expect that uniform to last long. Once you have decided to get serious about your studies you should invest in a medium-weight uniform. As you become more advanced you may want a heavy weight uniform simply because they stand up better to the type of treatment that you will be giving them.
2. Some schools are also open on Sunday's, but that is much less common.
3. Open sparring or training sessions so that you can simply go and spar and workout. Ideally your school is large enough that maybe there is a second training room so that a class can be taking place in one room and other students can be practicing in another room.
4. Does your school actually have martial arts seminars by visiting martial artists? Many schools claim that is a benefit. A school that I belonged to for nine years claimed this and never offered a single seminar during the entire nine years! (and we inquired repeatedly)
5. Competition program: if you're into that
6. Separate self-defense classes that focus on realistic scenarios and training methods
7. Separate weapons classes (generally for students who have been training for at least a year)
8. Demonstration team or a competition team to go to tournaments and demonstrations
9. Programs for younger students ages 4-6 (Little Ninjas, Junior Dragons or something like that) Generally these are Karate-like classes where children will usually wear a uniform and maybe earn a white belt but not study and actual curriculum. These programs are generally intended as a feeder to the regular programs and allow younger children to begin to learn some basic martial arts concepts and activities.
10. Generally it should be allowable to come in and practice whenever the school is open as long as there is a practice room or space toward the back of the main room to practice as long as you are not disturbing the class.

## *Monthly: Pay as You Go*

Monthly programs allow students to join and pay on a monthly basis without having to sign up for a one year or longer program. This provides flexibility so that if a student moves, changes schools or simply does not like the program a month or two into it; they are not stuck with a one-year membership. The disadvantage of this type of program is that over a longer period of time you will probably end up paying more than if you did sign up for a one year or longer program. There are always trade-offs.

If you sign up for some type of one year or longer program there will often be several payment methods:

### School Payment Methods

1. **MONTHLY:** Make an initial deposit followed by monthly payments until the program fee has been paid off. (interest will almost always be included)
2. **QUARTERLY:** Make four equal payments four months in a row and the program is paid off. Obviously these four payments are larger than the 12 monthly payments mentioned above.
3. **PAY-IN-FULL:** One lump sum payment for the entire one year program. Usually some type of discount (10%) might be offered if you are paying in full.

## *Contracts: What to Expect*

The first rule of contracts is **READ BEFORE YOU SIGN!** If you are not clear about what every single sentence in the contract means, get clarification so that you understand what you are getting into. Reading after you sign is too late!

Contracts will be written to provide the most flexibility and benefit for the school versus the student. That's simply how the business works. Read every line carefully and ask questions if you do not understand. Look for late fees, testing fees, belt fees, uniform costs, sparring equipment or any other requirements that might be part of the program. Find out if your program has a set time limit, such as one year, if it is possible to freeze the program. In other words, you may want to stop the clock for a few weeks if you know you will be out of town, or you become sick or injured or maybe just want a break without losing the time you have purchased. Often a program will say, for example, that you have one year or until you reach the rank of Blue Belt, whichever comes first. So if you are super dedicated like some students I have had, and earn your blue belt in six months, then your program is over and you have to sign up for the next level. On the other hand, if you spend a year training and you have not reached blue belt yet, your program is over. Either way this situation favors the school more than the student.

At United Karate, we did the opposite in order to favor the student. You could sign up for blue belt and you either had one year or you could continue to train beyond a year until you reached your blue belt. This positive policy actually resulted in more students staying with the program and ultimately accomplishing blue belt and continuing on to the black belt program. That is the goal of the school – retention of students. By favoring the students, you are actually favoring the school.

Schools will offer black belt programs and second degree black belt programs and masters or life programs. Each involves trade-offs which are based on whether you think you will stick with it or whether you are willing to make a long-term commitment. No one knows what the future holds. You may get transferred, become disabled, lose interest (ask if your program is transferable to another family member or someone else) or the school may go out of business. Not all martial arts schools are very financially stable. You will have to consider carefully which program suites your goals and tolerance for risk or uncertainty. (I sound like an investment advisor here, but that's what you're doing – making an investment).

## Location, Location, Location

You've heard that saying before. What I mean by this is that there are many locations or places to find a martial arts school. You may find a school at the YMCA, or within a sports club or a county recreation center. Your school may be located within a local strip mall shopping center or inside of a larger enclosed mall. It really does not matter where it is located as long as it is in a safe neighborhood and is a clean and reasonably spacious facility. I've already said this but it bears repeating, that you need to go watch several classes on several different occasions to see how they are run and how different instructors interact with students and how they control and motivate their classes.

## Costs

Martial arts are an art form, but they are also a business. Someone has to pay to keep the lights on. That being said, there are a variety of ways that schools generate revenue and keep the cash flowing in. This is not a bad thing, but you need to be aware of the various costs that you will likely incur on your journey.

### Martial Arts Costs and Fees

1. Uniform (good idea to have two)
2. Sparring gear. Padded head gear, mouth guard, hand, feet, shins and chest guard.
3. Testing fee (each belt level may require a test fee before you can graduate to the next belt level. This is in addition to your regular membership or program fee.
4. Seminar fees (unless they are included in the program contract)
5. Weapons (advanced students often purchase practice weapons such as foam nunchukas, or wood or bamboo swords or rubber knife or wooden gun for self-defense practice.
6. Tournament or competition fees (not generally part of your school)
7. If your school is part of a national or international affiliation such as the U.S. Tae Kwon Do Federation, or the World Tae Kwon Do Federation, then there may be separate annual membership fees or testing fees. Inquire about these fees or see if these are included in the membership at your school.
8. After school fees if you participate in one of these programs at the school.

## The Art of Shopping!

Now you are ready to begin your search. In the next few boxes below are a few key considerations when you visit a school:

### Tips for Visiting a School

1. Be respectful and polite. Respect is the first lesson in martial arts. Without it learning cannot take place.
2. Shake hands if an instructor offers to shake hands
3. If someone bows to you, bow back out of respect.
4. Call the school to find out if visitors are allowed to come and watch.
5. If there are high-pressure sales tactics, you don't want to be there.
6. Observe the classes quietly to show respect and not to distract the students or the instructors.
7. Do not try to impress anyone with what you have learned about martial arts in your reading. Focus on learning what you can.
8. Try to avoid discussing other schools you have visited; just focus on learning about the one you're in at the moment.
9. Classes will vary greatly from day to day and from instructor to instructor. Go observe many classes at the schools that seem to be on your short list. Every instructor has a bad day once in a while so watch enough classes to get a good idea. You may show up on a day when they are teaching weapons or self-defense only. The more classes you watch the better sampling you have to make your judgment.
10. Find out when enrollment is possible. Commercial schools will generally start any time. University programs or community centers will only start every six weeks or every semester. Check ahead of time.

I spoke wrote earlier about various styles of martial arts. There are also various ways of training in a given martial art. Below is a list of potential training styles that you should ask about to determine if the school teaches in a manner that is within your comfort zone. On the other hand, martial arts is about leaving your comfort zone and stretching your abilities to achieve new heights! But here's the list anyway:

## Training and Sparring Styles

1. Traditional – generally focusing on forms, kata, hyungs, poomse
2. Mixed Martial Arts – combination of various styles including boxing, grappling, wrestling and other striking arts – more or less the opposite of traditional
3. Sport Karate – involves light contact point sparring
4. Olympic-style – involves semi-contact
5. Full-contact – usually requires a tough personality and body
6. Self-Defense – focusing on realistic, practical street techniques without much study of an established martial art system

## School Atmosphere

1. Are students and instructors respectful toward each other?
2. Do the instructors appear to enjoy teaching or do they look like they can't wait for class to end?
3. Do students appear to be enjoying themselves?
4. Is the class fun but serious or is there too much joking around and silliness? It's ok to have some levity, but martial arts are a serious topic.
5. Do instructors pay attention to details; teaching concepts as well as the mechanics of a technique?

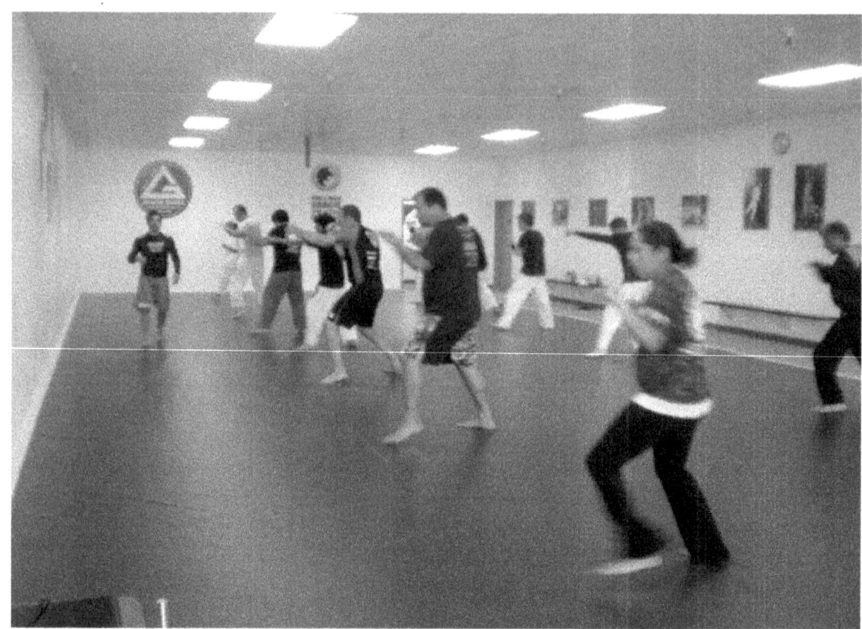

*A mixed martial arts class working out in their dojo*

## *The Best Style of Martial Art*

I am always amused when I hear someone ask what is the best style of martial art. There is no best martial art. They are all intended to focus on self-defense. The key is whether or not your training really focused on the reality of combat and self-defense in realistic scenarios and settings or just on memorization of forms/kata/hyungs/poomse and training for competition and sport karate.

If you do a Google search on "Bunkai" you will find that it is a Japanese term meaning interpretation of kata or forms. What 99% of martial arts schools teach in their kata is what really well versed martial artists refer to as the "B" knowledge. These are watered-down or made up explanations of how to use various moves from the kata. The kata or forms are simply the vocabulary of the given style. Like any language, you learn the vocabulary and basic structure and then you learn to write your own thoughts. In other words, on the street you would never jump in and begin to execute a green belt form, but you would use some of the moves from it (if you have studied the "A" knowledge through bunkai") to defend yourself.

A simple movement like a front-stance with a down-block is typically taught as blocking a roundhouse kick from your opponent. Try this for real and you will end up with a broken forearm. Which is stronger, your forearm or your opponent's shin? In reality a movement like that is intended to defend against someone who has grabbed your forearm. Step BACKWARDS, not forwards as you typically do in a kata, wrap around with the arm being grabbed and re-grab your opponent's forearm, while stepping back into your front stance, then down block against the back of their elbow as you drop your weight down suddenly into your front stance. The end result is your opponent has a broken or hyper extended elbow and will not be giving you any trouble for quite some time.

I realize this is difficult to visualize in written form, but the point is that every movement in a Tae Kwon Do form or any other form of any other style actually has three or four or many practical and often lethal applications if you spend enough time learning from someone who knows the kata. So take the movements you already know and study their practical application before going into another style of martial art and repeating the same behavior.

As far as other styles however, there are some that do come across a little more intuitive in the self-defense arena: Hapkido, Ed Parker Style Kenpo Karate, Jiu Jitsu, Krav Maga, to name a few. But again, any style can be effective if you are taught effectively. It depends up on how much knowledge you have about how to use the techniques you have learned.

***<u>When it comes to children</u>***, there are children who study Judo, Kendo (swordsmanship), various of the Chinese styles such as Wu Shu, Kung Fu and so forth. Clearly the most prevalent in the United States is Tae Kwon Do or one of the similar Japanese or Okinawan styles of Karate or Isshin Ryu (Ryu means school). What is good about these styles is that children can develop proficiency relatively easily and if they are taught with a self-defense emphasis as they get into their middle-school years, then they can apply these skills in a real situation if needed.

You must learn about many topics which I cover in my book ***"The Way of the Martial Artist"*** to be fully versed and prepared for self-defense whether it is in a parking lot or in Iraq. You must understand principles of camouflage, concealment and evasion. You must learn how to use your environment and terrain to your advantage. You must learn about weapons of opportunity; how to use what is at your disposal and within arm's reach to defend your self – and actually practice this vs. just reading about it. There are tactics and strategies and training methods that I discuss which will allow you to take what you have learned in the martial arts school and help you make it work in combat. That is the purpose of it all.

More important than any specific techniques are the proper knowledge, mindset and spirit. You must understand the real meanings of terms like timing and speed and how to isolate the difference between them in drills so that you can improve these qualities. You must develop a "survivor" mindset that also involves understanding of how you would truly react and what your triggers would be in a self defense situation. Where is your "line of conviction"? How far can someone push you before you react and then where will you enter into the force continuum. When we were operating our martial arts school United Karate Institute of Self Defense, Inc. we had a slogan that said it all:

***"If you can't defend yourself . . .***
***nothing else matters."***

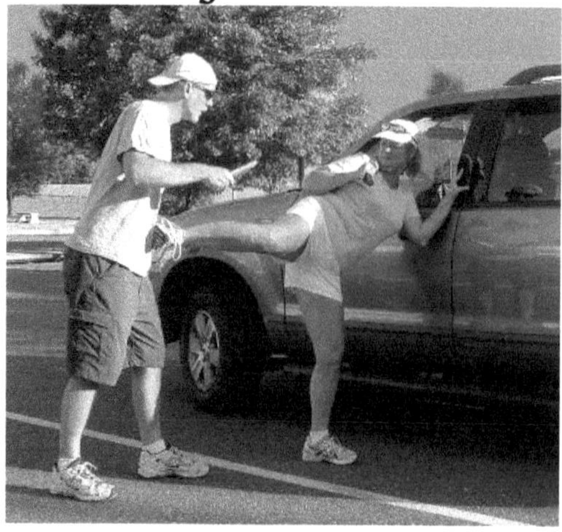

## *Shopping Around*

I have said many things about what to look for and what to expect from a martial arts school and your journey in the martial arts. There is no single school or instructor that will be perfect in every aspect. Do not think that because some aspects of a school, instructor or program may not meet every criteria perfectly that it is not a good school. Many schools will stack up about the same on any list of criteria or questions.

My goal is writing this book is the help you become familiar with what can be expected and what should be expected of you or your child so that you are a better educated student going into your martial arts experience. As you review this beginner's guide and visit schools and read about martial arts styles, you will become better at being able to differentiate between different schools and eventually make a good choice. Do not rush! Take your time so that you will find a school that will really be right for you. Re-read this book to review key points and then begin your search, but at some point, you must commit if you are ever going to begin your personal journey.

My experience has been that, generally speaking, many commercial schools are fairly similar in what they offer, what they cost and the quality of instruction that you receive. Some are considerably better in various areas and that is why you need to take your time and discover these differences.

You will need to do a lot of study on your own as you should in any academic or artistic endeavor. Read books, buy videos, surf the internet and check out martial arts magazines. There is much to learn and you will not find all of it at your school, but it should be your home base where you put into practice what you have learned. Do no rely on a single instructor to be your sole source of martial arts knowledge or training. There is too much out there to learn, experience and enjoy so don't limit yourself.

*Train hard and with good spirit.*
*You are the next generation of martial arts!*

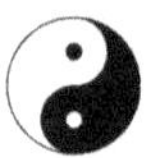

## Resources

**Books:**

1. Martial Arts for Dummies – Jenifer Lawler
2. The Complete Idiot's Guide to Martial Arts – Cezar Borkowski

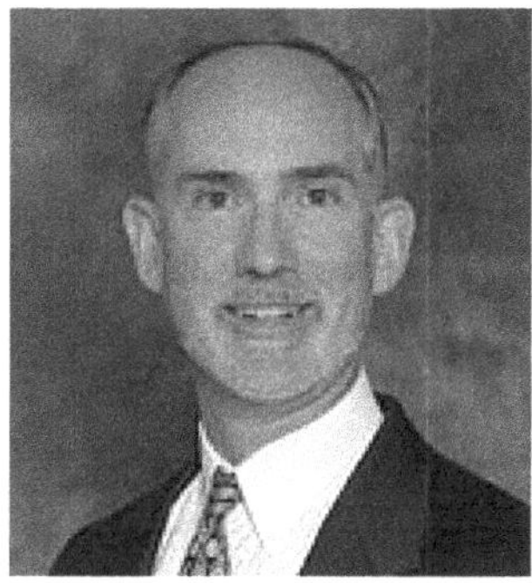

# About the Author

Kevin Brett is a certified martial arts instructor with twenty years of martial arts training and teaching experience. He and wife Lana Kaye Brett were two of the five co-founders of the United Karate Institute of Self-Defense, Incorporated in Alexandria, Virginia. He has taught martial arts and street self-defense to local law enforcement, military and federal officers focusing on realistic and practical application of martial arts techniques. He has studied Tae Kwon Do, Jiu Jitsu, Kendo, Kenjutsu, Kenpo Karate, Shotokan, Aiki Do and many other styles to add to his diverse experience base.

He is the President/CEO of Kevin Brett Studios, Inc., and the author of

- ***The Way of the Martial Artist: Achieving Success in Martial Arts and in Life!***
- ***Finding the Right Martial Arts School for You***
- ***Core Self-Defense: Personal Combat System***
- ***The Martial Arts Instructor Bible***

Information and samples from this comprehensive martial artist's guidebook can be viewed at www.KevinBrettStudios.com

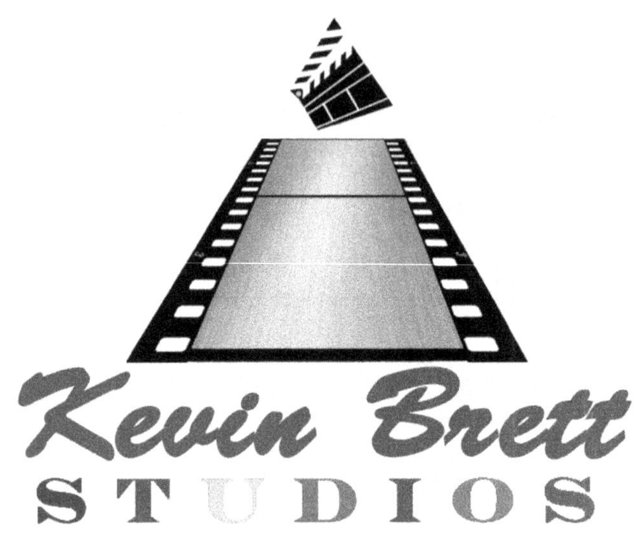
Kevin Brett
STUDIOS

# Appendix A: Listing of Internet Martial Arts School Directories

Below are the top ten martial arts school directories on the internet. Certainly a quick Google search can also help you find more schools in your area as well. Don't forget to check other possible avenues of locating a school as mentioned in the last chapter in the list titled "Where to Find Martial Arts Schools"

| Martial Arts School Directories |
|---|
| http://www.martialdirect.com/Category/Directory-Listings/ |
| http://www.dojos.com/directory.htm |
| http://www.dojolocator.com/ |
| http://www.masites.com/schools.cfm |
| http://www.martialinfo.com/search.asp |
| http://www.martialartslistings.com/ |
| http://www.usadojo.com/kata/schools.asp |
| http://www.martialartschoolsdirectory.com/ |
| http://www.martialedge.net/martial-arts-school-directory/ |
| http://www.martialschools.com/ |

# Appendix B: Dictionary of Common Martial Arts Terms

## Japanese Karate Ranking Systems

Most Japanese styles of Karate use a ranking system like the one below:

| Rank Name | Rank Degree or Belt Color |
|---|---|
| Judan | 10th degree black belt |
| Kudan | 9th degree |
| Hachidan | 8th degree |
| Shichidan | 7th degree |
| Rokudan | 6th degree |
| Godan | 5th degree |
| Yodan | 4th degree |
| Sandan | 3rd degree |
| Nidan | 2nd degree |
| Shodan | 1st degree |
| Ikkyu | 1st grade (1st brown belt) |
| Nikkyu | 2nd grade |
| Sankyu | 3rd grade |
| Yonkyu | 4th grade |
| Gokyu | 5th grade |
| Rokkyu | 6th grade |
| Shichikyu | 7th grade |
| Hachikyu | 8th grade |
| Kyukyu | 9th grade |
| Jukyu | 10th grade (white belt) |

## Chinese Ranking Systems

Chinese styles do not usually have a belt ranking system. In modern times, however, many Chinese style have adopted the custom of wearing a satin sash of various colors around the waist. These sashes can be black, red, silver, gold or white. However, the rank they denote varies from style to style.

| Male Titles | Founder of the System | Female Titles |
|---|---|---|
| Si-Tai Gung | Grandmaster | Si-Tai Poo |
| Si-Gung | Master | Si-Poo |
| Si-Bok | Instructor | Si-Do Goo |
| Si-Fu | Senior Instructor | Sifu |
| Si-Buk | Junior | Si-Goo Mui |
| Si-Hing | Older Classmate | Si-Je |
| Si-Di | Younger Classmate | Si-Mui |
| Sing-San (Husband) | Mate Outside of Art | Si-Mo (Wife) |
| Husband | | Wife |

## Korean Tae Kwon Do Ranking System

| Rank Name | Rank Degree or Belt Color |
|---|---|
| Shibdan | 10th degree black belt |
| Koodan | 9th degree |
| Paldan | 8th degree |
| Childan | 7th degree |
| Yookdan | 6th degree |
| Ohdan | 5th degree |
| Sandan | 4th degree |
| Samdan | 3rd degree |
| Yeedan | 2nd degree |
| Illdan | 1st degree |
| Ill Gup | Brown Belt |
| Yee Gup | Red Belt |

| San Gup | Purple Belt |
|---|---|
| Sa Gup | Blue Belt |
| Oh Gup | Dark Green Belt |
| Yuk Gup | Light Green Belt |
| Chi Gup | Orange Belt |
| Pal Gup | Yellow Belt |
| Koo Gup | White Belt |

Below are just a few of the styles of martial arts from Japan, China, Okinawa and Korea. Okinawan martial arts are often considered Japanese because of the close proximity of the two chains of islands. Wu Shu, Kung Fu, and Kenpo are some of the most widely recognized types of Chinese martial arts. There are many varieties of Kung Fu. Most styles of Kung Fu are divided between Northern Chinese styles and Southern Chinese styles. Below is table with just a few representative major styles of martial arts. It is important to realize that virtually every country from India to the Asian Pacific rim has many of its own styles as well. These below are just some of the better known styles.

| **Korean** | **Japanese** | **Chinese** | **Okinawan** |
|---|---|---|---|
| Taekyon | Aikido | Crane | Kobudo |
| Tae Kwon Do | Judo | Drunken | Karate |
| Tang Soo Do | Aiki-jujitsu | Monkey | Goju-ryu |
| Moo Duk Kwan | Goju-ryu | Eagle Claw | Issin-ryu |
| Yun Moo Kwan | Kyokushinai | Five Elders | Shorei-ryu |
| Chi Do Kwan | Shito-ryu | Hop Gar | Shorin-ryu |
| Oh Do Kwan | Shotokan | Ch'a Ch'uan | Shuri-te |
| Kuk Sool won | Wado-ryu | Hsing-I | |
| Hapkido | Kendo | Hsing-Yi | |
| Hwarang-do | Ninjitsu | Hung Ch'uan | |
| Subak | Kenjutsu | Leopard Style | |
| Chung Do Kwan | Iaido | Lion | |
| Chang Moo Kwan | Karate-Do | Monkey | |
| Song Moo Kwan | | Pa-Kua | |
| Ji Do Kwan | | Praying | |
| Kumdo | | Mantis | |
| | | White Crane | |
| | | Wing Chun | |
| | | Wu Shu | |
| | | Chin Na | |

| | | Dim Mak | |
|---|---|---|---|

## *Basic Tae Kwon Do Terms*

| Korean Word | English |
|---|---|
| Kyo Sah Nim | Instructor |
| Cha Ryut | Attention |
| Kyung-Nea | Bow |
| Jhoon-Bee | Ready |
| Si-Jak | Begin |
| Dedo-Dorah | About Face |
| Ko-Man or Goman | Stop |
| Ba-Ro | Return to Ready |
| Shio or Shuh | At Ease |
| Hyung or Poomse | Forms or Patterns |
| Ki-Hap | Tae Kwon Do Yell |
| Dobok | Uniform |
| Do-Jang | School or Workout Area |
| Sah-Bum-Nim | Chief Instructor (4th dan through 7th dan) |
| Kamsah-hom-ni-da | Thank you very much |
| Kimase | Horse stance |
| Jugoolse | Front stance |
| Fogoolse | Back stance |
| Ap Chagee | Front snap kick |
| Yup Chagee | Round kick |

| Korean Word | English |
|---|---|
| Ill | First |
| Yee | Second |
| Sam | Third |
| Sa | Fourth |
| Oh | Fifth |
| Yuk | Sixth |
| Chil | Seventh |
| Pal | Eighth |
| Ku | Ninth |
| Sip | Tenth |
| Chagee | Kicks |
| Daeryun | Sparring |
| Jayne Daeryun | Free sparring |
| Knifehand | Soodo |
| Hoshinsool | Self defense techniques |

| Kyuk Pa | Breaking |
|---|---|
| Ha-na | One |
| Tul | Two |
| Set | Three |
| Net | Four |
| Ta-Sot | Five |
| Yo-Sot | Six |
| Il-Ghop | Seven |
| Yo-Dul | Eight |
| A-Ho | Nine |
| Yuhl | Ten |

# Appendix C: Goal Setting and Planning Worksheet

The worksheet below was built with just a simple spreadsheet. The format is not important except that you want it to be readable and easy to use. Design your own. Have a separate tab for each month to track progress and then maybe a new spreadsheet for each year to keep track of your near-term, medium-term and long-term goals, progress, notes, concerns and accomplishments. For planning purposes, the worksheet below captures all of the key elements of setting and planning goals. Build your own and get started! If you are serious, then write down your goals and be specific about what, why, when, how and so forth. Make your plan for success now. Good luck!

## Goal Setting and Planning Worksheet

For each goal, think it through and describe it in as much detail as you can.

| | Long Term Goals (10 years) | Start Date | End Date | Why do you want to achieve this goal? Why is it important? |
|---|---|---|---|---|
| 1 | | | | |
| 2 | | | | |
| 3 | | | | |

| | Long Term Qualities - list 3 qualities that will help you accomplish this goal | | Progress toward your goals |
|---|---|---|---|
| 1 | | Goal 1 | |
| 2 | | Goal 2 | |
| 3 | | Goal 3 | |

| | Medium Term Goal (5 years) | Start Date | End Date | Why do you want to achieve this goal? Why is it important? |
|---|---|---|---|---|
| 1 | | | | |
| 2 | | | | |
| 3 | | | | |

| | Medium Term Qualities - list 3 qualities that will help you accomplish this goal | | Progress toward your goals |
|---|---|---|---|
| 1 | | Goal 1 | |
| 2 | | Goal 2 | |
| 3 | | Goal 3 | |

| | Near Term Goals (6-12 months) | Start Date | End Date | Why do you want to achieve this goal? Why is it important? |
|---|---|---|---|---|
| 1 | | | | |
| 2 | | | | |
| 3 | | | | |

| | Near Term Qualities - list 3 qualities that will help you accomplish this goal | | Progress toward your goals |
|---|---|---|---|
| 1 | | Goal 1 | |
| 2 | | Goal 2 | |
| 3 | | Goal 3 | |

| Obstacles to Achieving My Goals<br><br>These are gaps in my abilities, skills, resources, knowledge training, social connections, finances, physical fitness | Who Can Help Me?<br><br>Family members, friends, coaches, mentors |
|---|---|
| | |
| | |
| | |
| | |
| | |
| | |

# Index

# O



# P



# Q



# R



# S



# T



# U



# V



# W



# Z

www.ingramcontent.com/pod-product-compliance
Lightning Source LLC
Chambersburg PA
CBHW070954040426
42443CB00007B/496

* 9 7 8 0 9 8 1 9 3 5 0 4 1 *